Painful Dilemma

William Campbell Douglass II, MD

Painful Dilemma

ISBN 9962-636-00-0

Cover illustration by
María Luisa Gutiérrez
and
Alex Manyoma (alex@3dcity.com)

Please, visit Rhino's website for other publications from
Dr. William Campbell Douglass
www.rhinopublish.com

Dr. Douglass' "Real Health" alternative medical newsletter is
available at www.realhealthnews.com

RHINO PUBLISHING, S.A.
World Trade Center
Panama, Republic of Panama

Voicemail/Fax
International: + 416-352-5126
North America: 888-317-6767

Painful Dilemma

PATIENTS IN PAIN
PEOPLE IN PRISON

William Campbell Douglass II, MD

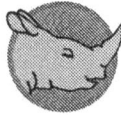

Rhino Publishing, S.A.

Pain has an Element of Blank
It cannot recollect
When it begun or if there were
A time when it was not

It has no Future but itself
Its Infinite contain
Its Past enlightened to perceive
New Periods of Pain.

Emily Dickinson, Circa I862 – 1890

INTRODUCTION:

<u>At any given moment, one in every six adult Americans is in pain</u>. About 40% of Americans experience headaches regularly. Back pain and arthritis affect about 50 million people. As the older population increases, the number of people in pain increases. These figures do not include the millions suffering pain from cancer, peripheral vascular disease, trauma, neurological diseases and others. Pain, no matter the source, is our number one complaint.

GENERAL COMMENTS

Everybody has suffered from pain — especially the intense acute pain that flares up when the nail of a finger is hit with a hammer instead of the nail in the board or when a finger is burned on a pan along with the steak. That pain soon goes away even though the suffering can be intense. <u>But at least 20 million Americans</u> suffer from chronic pain that lasts for weeks or months -- or never goes away until the Grim Reaper wraps his comforting arms around the wretched victim. Most of its sufferers are the middle-aged and the elderly, <u>especially</u> the elderly. Lucky indeed are those who die in their sleep.

The most common form of chronic pain in the industrialized West is low back pain, which arises from osteoarthritis, ligament strains from improper lifting or other causes, and is estimated to afflict <u>15 percent of the population</u>. Cancer patients often suffer severe pain as their condition worsens. This is usually due to an expanding tumor encroaching on nerve fibers. It can be a pain from hell. Burn victims may have excruciating pain during recovery. Chronic pain includes tension and migraine headaches. Individuals with arthritis often suffer from chronic pain. The pain of arthritis isn't as excruciating as the pain of nerve compression or the pain of intestinal inflammation of the peritoneal variety but it is, nonetheless, debilitating and depressing.

Chronic pain is one of the nation's most costly health problems. <u>The price tag each year comes to nearly $50 billion for medical costs, lost income, lost productivity, compensation payments and legal costs.</u>

To the individual, the impact can be devastating both personally and professionally. Severe pain can impair sleep and appetite, and it can trigger anxiety, frustration and depression. Over time, pain can lower self-esteem ("I'm just a bother to everyone and have no useful purpose — I wish I were dead.") Pain does destroy the will to live. It destroys the sex drive. As long as there is neglected pain, there will be Kevorkians to offer the Ultimate Solution.

Until recently, pain management, especially chronic pain management, was seldom included in medical curricula. In fact, pain was, and still generally is, considered «an essential part of the human experience.» Those who bear the greatest pain are admired and accorded great respect. You are of a higher moral order and your courage is a sign of your manliness, whichever your sex. Fortunately, that attitude is changing.

Because pain is so personal and subjective, medical teaching has generally chosen to work around it by calling it a «necessary evil.» Pain helps the doctor to make a diagnosis; it is often the early warning sign of a serious and life-threatening emergency. However, in four years of medical school, we did not have <u>one hour</u> devoted to the subject of treating pain, or even how to make the patient comfortable. Granted that making the patient comfortable is primarily the job of the nursing staff, however it's the doctor's responsibility as well. He is the one who made the deep gash in the patient's belly to repair the aneurysm, bored the holes in his head to relieve a subdural hematoma, or amputated his crushed arm at the elbow. <u>These procedures hurt</u> and the "necessary evil" is no longer necessary. The scientific modalities are there to prevent this suffering.

PERCEPTIONS OF PAIN

An expert on pain recently stated in an article in Scientific American: "As common as it is, pain can be extremely elusive. The patient may have difficulty describing it, and the physician often cannot substantiate it. An individual in acute pain may scream and writhe in agony; but the person with chronic pain often appears outwardly normal, with few visible signs. This makes it difficult for the doctor and the patient."

If the doctor can not substantiate the pain by palpation of the affected part or by X-ray or other "scientific" means, he immediately becomes suspicious and defensive: Is this patient just looking for attention? Is he an addict? Is he crazy?

I know all about these mental mechanisms. As a young doctor, I reacted the same way. And that was long before the present drug paranoia when you could prescribe all the narcotic you felt the patient needed with no questions asked. Those were indeed the Good Old Days from the patient's point of view, at least to a point. But we were all afflicted with the fear of addiction, drug tolerance and respiratory depression and so, although better than today's paralysis in the field of pain relief, it was less than perfect and many patients suffered terribly because of our ignorance <u>and unfounded fears of addiction</u>.

Pain is difficult for the patient to describe and the physician to evaluate. Although much remains to be learned about the mechanism of pain, we know individuals have different levels of tolerance to pain. There are also differences in individual sensitivity to drugs, and in how drugs are metabolized. Studies indicate that pain relief from opiates varies by age, race, cultural differences, type of pain and location of pain. Because the effectiveness of pain medication varies greatly from person to person, <u>a patient's need for a high dose is not necessarily a sign of addiction</u>.

With the same affliction, some people hurt more than others. It will not do to consider them weak, childish or stupid just because they experience more pain than what you think is "proper" for that illness. As a young doctor, I didn't understand this; pain was pain and that's all there was to it. It seemed obvious, even to my young brain, that all pains were not equal but I thought each type of pain should be more or less the same in each person. You learn otherwise after you have experienced a little pain yourself. Maybe no one under the age of 50 should be allowed to take care of pain patients. A little personal experience in the field of pain is a great teacher.

Which experiences pain the most, men or women? Many studies suggest that women report or feel pain more acutely than men, and are more likely to report to a pain center for treatment. However, it's not clear if the difference is due to women actually experiencing more pain, or sociologic, with men less likely to admit they are having a problem — the old stiff-upper-lip attitude.

Studies have shown that women perceive taste sensations, such as sweet, sour, bitter or salty, at lower levels of concentration than men, i.e., they are more sensitive to these stimuli. They can more easily detect an electrical stimulus as well. This difference is heightened during the luteal phase of menstruation, the time just after ovulation. While studies on pain perception have had conflicting results, laboratory research suggests that women do also have a lower tolerance to pain or, put another way, are more sensitive to pain. Some studies have shown that if women are supplemented with oral contraceptives during the luteal phase of the menstrual cycle, the threshold for pain is the same as for males. This isn't absolutely proven, this relationship of hormones to pain sensitivity, because the studies were small.

And the smell sensitivity of women, in my experience, is quite remarkable compared to men. They must have olfactory nerves twice the size of ours. During a period when I was experiencing bad breath from an undetected abscessed tooth, my daughter could detect that I hadn't cleaned my teeth from across the room — "Daddy, you've been eating sheep dung again!" Enough about women and on to children.

Pain in and of itself can be hazardous, whether or not an infant remembers the sensation. Pain increases the heart rate, blood pressure and stress hormones, and a 1992 study found that babies undergoing surgery had less morbidity, mortality, and complications if they were given a deep anesthetic compared to light sedation. Some people just don't seem to think babies are human (in or out of the womb.) If you are going to have your little guy circumcised — and I do not recommend it — make the doctor promise to use a local anesthetic. More on children and pain later.

As I was writing this report, yet another pain study was reported in the lay press. The headline of the article gave the gist of the depressing story:

Hospitals Failing Post-op Pain Relief

The conclusion I was compelled to reach in this monograph will come as a surprise to many of my friends and readers. Quite candidly, it came as a surprise to me as well. I set out to write about the serious problem of pain and neglect of this problem by a large portion of the medical profession. Along the way, however, I was struck by two important and unavoidable facts:

(1) Many physicians and medical researchers mistakenly believe that their primary goal is to prolong life and

(2) The so-called "war on drugs" is not only a failure but it has led to the prolongation of pain in patients whose only crime was to become seriously ill.

On (1) above, this life-extending assumption underlies the constant media references to the increasing life span of Americans — pain has gotten lost in the obsession over life extension. Who wants to live to be 90 if they are in pain? <u>The success of Dr. Kevorkian is 90 percent a reaction to unremitting pain</u>. With the successful treatment of pain, Dr. Kevorkian would be just another obscure pathologist. The doctor's primary goal is the <u>relief of suffering,</u>

not life extension. Certainly we should work to extend life but, as I see it, that's primarily God's job. I don't see any evidence that "ever-lasting life" is meant to be on this planet, unless you are Buddhist.

I urge you to read the pieces in the Appendix. They are not there just to add weight to the book. If you don't like appendices, at least read Appendix IV for some words of wisdom on the «drug war» by a distinguished jurist, Senior Judge: *John L. Kane of the U.S. District Court of Denver, Colorado: The War on Drugs: An Impossible Dream.*

As you will see in the pages that follow, and as many of you know from firsthand experience, a life in pain is no life at all. Pain consumes you: sapping your physical strength, exhausting your mental energy and crushing your spirit.

PART I

PATIENTS IN PAIN

There are many drugs to eliminate pain and they are, for the most part, narcotics. But this does not mean they should be linked with "street drugs" such as crack, pot and heroin. The street drugs are indeed derivatives of narcotics or amphetamine but they are usually contaminated and taken in very large doses for mind alteration, not pain relief.

Here's the popular view about pain relief from an associated Press writer:

"The man was dying of lung cancer. For a while, morphine controlled his severe chest pain. But eventually, inevitably, the cancer began literally suffocating him. His panic grew as his breathing labored. More morphine could relieve that horrible feeling of smothering, but with a risk: It also could further reduce respiration. The doctor gave his patient enough morphine to ease his suffering. Later that day, the man died peacefully, his family at his side." (Associated Press, 10/15/99)

There is an innuendo here, just below the surface: The doctor quietly and skillfully killed the patient with a little too much morphine, right in front of the family.

"How much pain medication to give terminally ill patients, when the medication itself might hasten death, long has been a quandary," the reporter added.

The tragedy here is two-fold: First, doctors out of fear of killing the patient through respiratory depression, let the patients suffer, and second, this 19th century horror happens because of a lack of understanding by doctors of how narcotics work in terminally ill patients. Even the few doctors who do understand are afraid of incurring the wrath of ignorant medical boards and legislators who do not – and so patients die in pain.

A study in 1998 found one in four elderly cancer patients in nursing homes received <u>no treatment at all</u> for daily pain. If there is one message I would like to impart to my colleagues, if I knew I had only one more shot left to fire, it would be:<u> "IN THE 21st CENTURY, IT IS NO LONGER NECESSARY FOR PATIENTS TO ENDURE PAIN. YOU MUST FIGHT FOR THE PATIENT'S RIGHT NOT TO SUFFER -- CURE IS NOT ALWAYS POSSIBLE; FREEDOM FROM PAIN IS."</u>

Research has been reported in respected journals, such as Lancet, that giving adequate pain relief, even with large doses of morphine, does not shorten the lives of terminally ill patients. Some health professionals have criticized the practice, comparing it to euthanasia, but doctors at St. Christopher's Hospice in London claim patients receiving higher doses of drugs such as morphine live just as long as those who do not. This has been reported many times. <u>There is no excuse for letting terminally ill patients die in pain.</u> The issue is settled. Everyone seems to know that except the doctors.

"This study dispels the myth that good pain control at the end of life means killing the patient. People should not fear that taking morphine for pain need shorten life, and any doctor with such a worry about one of their patients should seek specialist palliative care advice," said Nigel Sykes, one of the authors of the Lancet study, in a report to Reuters News. (That "worrying doctor" should also take a course in pain management. If you can't relieve suffering, you are not a complete doctor.) "There is no connection between competent symptom control and euthanasia," Dr. Sykes added.

Ref:
    Lancet, 7/28/00
    Reuters, 7/28/00

There is a ray of hope. At least 15 states recently have passed laws ensuring doctors' licenses won't be revoked for prescribing powerful controlled substances, like morphine, for severe pain. I started fighting to repair this out-

rageous blind spot in medicine five years ago.
But, in many ways things only got worse. Now,
the walls of ignorance and fear are beginning to
crumble.

The American Hospital Association (AHA)
declared in August, 1999, that all patients have a
right to proper pain management. Can you imagine, in the 21st Century, America's hospitals
having to make a statement like that? Well anyway, it happened -- maybe just in time for you,
IF you have a serious accident and IF the doctors are listening.

PAIN CONTROL GETS NATIONAL ATTENTION

Another organization with more and larger
teeth than the AHA has joined the war against
pain. The Joint Commission on the Accreditation of Healthcare Organizations is scoring
hospitals and other healthcare entities on how
well they assess and treat pain in all patients.
"The [new pain] standards are necessary because pain is a major public health issue in this
country," Janet McIntyre, spokeswoman for the
commission, told WebMD.

For Susan Wolf, 42, a North Carolina resi-
dent who suffers from rheumatoid arthritis, this
rush to sanity didn't come soon enough. She
told WebMD reporter Sean Martin about her
1996 knee replacement operation: "I woke up
from surgery in agony. The doctors refused to
help. I'll never forget -- there were men in white
coats with their arms crossed looking down at

me saying, 'We cannot do anything else. We're not allowed to give you more than x amount of drugs per hour.' I was lying there crying and in horrible pain. I ended up staying in the hospital longer than the doctor had initially said I would. And my recovery took a lot longer and was more difficult."

Susan Wolf's experience is common but there are many situations where the roles are <u>exactly reversed</u> -- the doctor, recognizing the genuine nature of the pain, prescribes adequate narcotic but the patient leaves the pills in the drawer for fear of addiction.

I have a friend, age 25, who was a UPS driver. She had severe accident on the way to a delivery. It was so severe that she had to have a fusion of two of her neck bones. Because of her neck pain, she can not sleep and so she is severely disabled. The doctor has given her adequate narcotic medication but she refuses to take it for fear of addiction.

I have explained to her that she is <u>inhibiting her recovery</u> by not giving her body a rest from pain. I even gave her pertinent parts of this manuscript to read (I knew she wouldn't read the entire book; most people don't read books) proving that pain relief is a <u>vital part of the recovery process</u>. It's similar to the SP block I have mentioned frequently in this desideratum. When the pain gateway in the neck is closed by an SP ganglion block with liquid cocaine, the headache, for example, will often be permanently cured because the body has had a chance to regroup and affect a recovery.

Will she take my advice? I think there is a fifty-fifty chance that she will overcome her narcophobia because she is sick of being sick.

According to Leeann Rhodes, MD, medical director of pain management at Washington Hospital Center (DC), "If you have a patient's pain under control, they are going to get up and [recover] better, they're going to be able to eat better, and their whole quality of life is better. If they have physical therapy, they will be more compliant." Hippocrates redux -- and a good thing too.

Joint Commission spokesperson, McIntyre said: "If you have breast cancer, you not only have to be treated for your breast cancer, but for any pain that might be associated with that cancer…The whole idea is recognizing that pain management is a crucial component of quality care." Isn't it amazing that a truism like that has to be articulated? Adequate pain relief has been available for at least 100 years but, better late than never -- right?

At Washington Hospital Center, Dr. Rhodes says: "At least every 8 hours, inpatients have their pain rated. ... Every time an outpatient comes through one of our clinics, the pain is rated. Zero is no pain. Ten is the worst pain im- aginable. It is what the patient says, not what the physician or nurse feels that the pain rating should be."

Last year, the commission first measured hospitals' pain programs, but didn't score them for accreditation. This year, the grades will count in whether a hospital keeps its accreditation. <u>THAT</u> will get their attention a lot faster than pronouncements from the AHA and all the ululations and moaning of the entire patient population put together. Power and money (same thing) talks -- gentle persuasion walks.

Susan Wolf, the patient who had to endure excruciating pain and humiliation following her knee operation --"We can't give you anything else for pain." -- is skeptical. She thinks hospitals will have difficulty complying because of doctor resistance to this simple humanitarian effort being imposed from above. In Susan's words: "...the medical culture has given pain care short shrift." But, she admitted, "We have come a long way in five years."

"In allowing treatment of chronic ... pain to be included as a 'patients' rights' issue, physicians may be pressured to prescribe opiates in cases in which this is inappropriate," wrote San Gorgonio Memorial Hospital's George Hansen, MD, in a letter to The Journal of the American Medical Association. "Patients with chronic pain are at substantial risk for drug abuse and addiction."

Get with it, George; you're practicing in the 21st Century; Freud is dead; <u>people in pain do not become addicted</u>. Listen to Richard Frankenstein, MD, a JCAHO official, who responded to your tragically outmoded view: "Flawed conceptions about addiction, tolerance, and dependence ... must be dispelled."

This myth of addiction in pain patients has been dispelled for the umpteenth time in a study published last April, 2000 in The Journal of the American Medical Association (JAMA): <u>an increased use of morphine for pain control during the past decade did not cause increased drug abuse</u>.

In the JAMA study, David E. Joranson and colleagues at the University of Wisconsin Medical School in Madison found that medical prescriptions for morphine-like drugs <u>increased</u> from 1990 to 1996. However, cases involving abuse of these drugs <u>dropped</u> from just over 5% of all drug abuse cases to 3.8% during the same time period.

<u>Joranson concluded in his WebMD interview: "The major implication of our study is that there is no support for the fear that opioid abuse would increase if the appropriate medical use of opioids increases.</u>"

If we can just keep up this momentum, your next operation should be a cake walk.

Ref: WebMD Washington Correspondent, Sean Martin, 1/12/01

****

In November, 1999, Oregon's medical board became the first to ever discipline a doctor for under treating pain. Among the complaints was that the doctor only provided Tylenol for a dying and suffering cancer patient. One pain specialist put the issue in focus: "...Pain is the issue, not preservation of life."

Some doctors fear that the current Federal legislation could reverse the progress being made at the state level. The federal legislation would formally declare prescribing controlled substances to alleviate pain a legitimate medical decision even if those drugs increase risk of death.

This problem should continue to be addressed at the state level. DRIGA, the Douglass Rule of Inverse Government Action, will probably come into play: "The more the government tries to relieve a problem, the worse the problem gets." The above wording in the proposed Federal law seems to be a tacit approval of euthanasia: "... even if those drugs increase the risk of death."

See what I mean? No matter what they legislate, being for the most part ignoramuses and a parliament of whores, they will complicate things and thus make the situation worse. What they need to do is abolish all of the drug laws, which are unconstitutional anyway, and demand that the president and his in-house goons, from the FBI to the BATF, cease and desist from this war against the American people and especially the heartless withholding of narcotics from people suffering pain. Which leads to my second conclusion...

My second conclusion is a touchier subject and I am (again) not being politically correct. The charade called "the war on drugs" has not stopped the flow or the use of street drugs but it has stolen many of our constitutional rights, has allowed the federal and state governments to increase their police power over innocent, law-abiding Americans and it has all but taken away the doctor's best weapon against pain. On the stripping away of our rights, consider this: Mr. Clinton gave (without any constitutional authority) the right to federal agents to do "sweeps" of federal housing projects for guns.

Ultimately then, the most effective way to eliminate the suffering of millions of innocent people is to get the government out of the drug enforcement business. More people are living off the drug enforcement industry than the number of people taking drugs illegally.

Allow me to relate to you a particularly gruesome story about the persecution of a doctor by state, not federal authority, for helping patients in pain from terminal illness. You must realize that the attacks on your liberties are coming from two police/legislative bodies --

The federal (legislative, judicial and executive branches) and the <u>state</u>. The states of New York and California, for instance, <u>are more Nazi-like than the federal government itself</u>. However, even the relatively free states, such as Utah, have put on the jack boots and black uniforms to "war" against drugs, as you will see.

Robert Weitzel MD, ran a headache clinic in Salt Lake City, the city that was founded so the Mormons could escape federal persecution. Well now, the state of Utah is laying on the persecution with both hands.

Armed agents of the state entered the office unannounced and confiscated 80 urine samples to test for narcotic content. Every sample was clear of any narcotic trace. But the witch hunt was on with interrogation of patients, riffling of files and minute inspection of the doctor's trash.

You may not know it, but many doctors are paid prostitutes for state and federal prosecutors. For a $25,000 fee they can get a specialist, in any field, to say whatever they want him to say. Add the threat that failure to cooperate may lead to an IRS investigation and/or an investigation of their practice methods, and every one of these despicable doctors will crow to the jury outrageous opinions on medical matters they do not understand. In the Weitzel case, their hired harlot testified that the care given constituted "active euthanasia." Exhumation of three of the deceased patients in 1999 revealed no detectable levels of morphine in two of them and a dose commensurate with normal practice in the third one.

Defense medical witnesses <u>completely contradicted</u> the testimony of the state's paid canary and stated that "... the terminally-ill patients received appropriate care...and that the time of the administration of the opiates <u>bore no rational relationship to the time of death</u>."

It was, clearly, an open-and-shut case for acquittal. So even the prosecutors were stunned when the jury returned a verdict of guilty to two counts of manslaughter. The doctor was sentenced to one to 15 years in prison.

There is an important lesson here for all of us. Perhaps you have already learned it the hard way, as I did. The jury system no longer serves the prosecution and the defense; it only serves the prosecution. The exception to this is the trial of bums, common thieves and the lower classes of all races. Since the 1960s, when the ACLU agitated for a relaxation of qualifications for jury duty, the juries have been composed of the lowest common denominator of our society, for the most part, well-meaning, uneducated, ignoramuses. One juror said to the press, after the Weitzel trial: "Gee, I didn't know he would go to prison." There was a lot he didn't know and the lesson here is: If you face prosecution, and you have a college degree, or make more than $100,000 a year, <u>settle out of court</u> if at all possible. It's hard to win when the court system has become to look like those tribunals of the French revolution.

[I am indebted to AAPS News (May, 2001), the newsletter of the Association of American Physicians and Surgeons, for revealing this case to their members. Dr. Weitzel is bankrupt and unemployed. He has won a new trial and desperately needs help. You can help by contacting Peter Waldo, Esq. 9 Exchange Place, Suite 1000, Salt Lake City, UT 84111.]

And so my conclusion is: <u>We must put an end to government intrusion by legalizing drugs</u>. (I can't believe I said that.) In so doing, we will, I hope, recover our constitutional rights and stop the shocking police state methods now being employed, as often as not, against innocent Americans: illegal surveillance, seizure of property without warrant or evidence, arbitrary arrests and, perhaps the most frightening of all, the federalization and militarization of our local police forces. As a result, we now have a standing army among us -- the very thing our forefathers warned us against.

I came to this conclusion on legalization after much research, prayer and soul-searching. I hope you will see, as I have, that the "war on drugs" has been a sham from the beginning. I would like to hear your reaction to this book. <u>Tell me where I'm wrong</u>. We're all seeking answers to a chimera with two ugly heads -- a police state tyranny that's destroying our country and a tyranny of street drugs that is also destroying our country. I expect to get a truckload of mail on this one and I will not be able to answer your letter but I promise to read all of them and I will make some general replies in the "Letters" column of my medical newsletter, REAL HEALTH -- (www.realhealthnews.com or call toll free: 1-800-851-7100).

But, ultimately, this book is about pain and it is my fervent desire, as someone whose life has been occupied relieving pain, that you will, after reading these pages, have a clearer perspective on the problems of competing interests between the government, the doctors and the patients who are caught in the middle of this painful dilemma.

Albert Schweitzer once said: "We must all die. But if I can save him from days of torture, that is what I feel is my great and ever new privilege. Pain is a more terrible lord of mankind than even death itself."

Douglass Aphorism Number VI : "Life without pain is a truly wonderful thing." That's not as elegant as Dr. Schweitzer's statement but it's true that most of us don't appreciate Freedom From Pain until we are seized by the Pain Monster in some part of our body and are thus rendered incommunicado, incoherent, incontinent, impotent and even pushed to the penultimate escape mechanism: inchoate insanity. When pain takes over, life is consumed by one goal -- avoidance of pain. Yet, only recently, have some modern doctors turned their attention to this part of their Hippocratic Oath: the relief of suffering from pain. Please note that I said some, and a minority at that.

That famous philosopher, pederast and humorist, Woody Allen, gave us one of the great one-liners of the 20th Century: "I'm not afraid of dying; I just don't want to be there when it happens." I have my own one-liner on the subject of dying (Douglass Aphorism Number One): "Everybody wants to go to heaven but nobody wants to die." But we are both a little off the mark on this one and the common denominator of our error is -- PAIN. If one is in the grip of unremitting pain of an exquisite nature, and there is no hope for relief, death is eagerly embraced and many a tomb stone should have engraved upon it : "Finally, a good night's sleep."

SOME HISTORY OF PAIN

You may not like history. I hated it in high school. But this is the <u>history of pain</u>. It's part of the human condition and part of your life experience -- whether you like it or not. <u>Pain can be funny</u> -- honest; it really can. Read on and you will see.

Throughout history, pain and medicine have gone hand-in-hand. This is obviously a truism but attitudes toward pain change with the times, not only the doctor's attitude but that of the patient. The flagellants of the Middle ages, for instance, tormented themselves in ways that seem preposterous today. They would not only inflict blows upon themselves with chains but apply red-hot coals and branding irons to their bodies. Napoleon's soldiers, during the Russian campaign, would have a limb amputated and then go back into battle on horseback. In the Good Old Days in India, if you were lucky, you could have yourself pierced through the abdomen and hung to swing on a hook. By doing this, you were contributing to an abundant harvest and increasing the fertility of the people.

From these jolly times we have inherited the expression, "getting off the hook." Pain is not so hard to endure when it is being inflicted upon someone else, especially if it is helping the crops and promoting fecundity.

Before the 20th Century, surgical incisions almost always became infected. The doctors thought it was part of the healing process and called it "laudable pus." As with pus, during much of the history of medicine, pain has been considered a necessary part of the healing process, -- "laudable pain," so to speak. In ancient Greece, if you were a criminal, the odds were you would not die an easy death. You would get lots of pain -- and it would not be laudable. Anatomists Herophilus and Erasistratus were given live criminals by the king from the dungeons for dissection "so they might capture in the raw what nature had kept hidden from them..." (The History of Pain, Rey, Harvard University Press, 1999)

Some physicians in "the age of enlightenment" believed in "laudable pain" to the extent that they would inflict pain in order to cure it! They would use cautery, friction, flagellation and urtication. These various forms of torture "would provoke a beneficial discharge and awakening sensibility." One of the most popular methods to fight pain with pain was "moxibustion," which consisted of a stiff fabric "stick" with vegetable fibers in it. This burning concoction was placed on the skin "to create a diversionary point." It was quite effective in diverting the pain so other doctors embraced it enthusiastically. The name of this medical genius is lost in the haze of antiquity.

Even in ancient times, not all doctors were indifferent to pain and suffering. In the first century, the Greek physician and naturalist, Dioscorides, suggested the root of the mandragora plant steeped in wine be given to patients before flesh or limbs were cut. The Roman naturalist Pliny reported that mandragora, also called the "potion of the condemned," was used to reduce the pain of crucifixion. Crucifixion is not popular anymore but fashions change and so, you just never know. But whether crucifixion makes a comeback or not, pain is pain and the mandragora plant is worth investigation.

Mandrake, or mandrogora, is a native to southeastern Europe and the Mediterranean. The ancients used Mandrake root to relieve pain and promote sleep, but it was also known to cause strange delirium and madness. The leaves are harmless and cooling when used as a poultice. Mandrake is the object of many strange superstitions: "It groweth beneath the gallows of murderers." And: "To digge the root bringeth sure deathe, as the shrieks emitting thenceforth can be herde by no man and live. It is therefore recommended to tie a dogge to the root, so that by struggling to free himself the plant may be dislodged without human hurte."

Aretaeus of Cappadocia, who lived in Rome in 100, AD, was an exceptionally fine physician in that his descriptions of diseases were remarkably accurate and still apply to this day. But on the treatment side he was a victim of his times, having little to work with. For migraine headache, for instance, he would first do bloodletting of the arm and then the forehead. Then the head was shaved and hot towels were applied to prepare the shaved head for scarification and cupping (more blood loss). Then to stop the bleeding, a branding iron was applied to the head wounds. (I wonder how many Florents they paid for that stimulating therapy.) When all this failed, the old reliable trephination was used. There's nothing like a hole in the head, according to the experts of the time, to relieve your headache.

The ancient Egyptians had invented this clever therapy thousands of years earlier.

Speaking of the popular branding iron, a famous surgeon, Hermann Boerhaave, who had a disease syndrome named after him, was in favor of the frequent use of the red-hot iron, especially in cases of hysteria and convulsions, which, apparently, he considered to be psychological. He was convinced that just the threat of the branding iron "would be enough to suppress all such symptoms of disorder" -- and I'll bet it worked.

Dioscorides, who lived in the time of Aretaeus mentioned above, was very familiar with narcotics 1900 years ago. One gets the impression, from reading the history of those times that, like today, narcotics were not used as extensively as they should have been. Among the pain-killers available were the opium poppy, the field poppy, marijuana, alcohol, lettuce, belladonna, henbane and black nightshade.

Marijuana, you may be surprised to learn, has been used in medicine for five-thousand years. Marijuana is mentioned five times in the Bible under such names as kaneh or kannabus which is translated into "aromatic cane" or "sweet cane." The first three mentions in the Bible (Exodus 30:22-23; Song of Songs 4:4-14; Isaiah 43:23-24) are highly favorable to its use. The last two (Jeremiah 6:20; Ezekiel 27:19) are neutral if not negative. Yahweh's adherents favored cannabis, another name for marijuana, as did the worshipers of the Hebrew god, Ashteroth or Astarte, known as "Queen of Heaven," "Star of the Sea," and "Stella Maris." (Now that sounds like a pot-smoking goddess, doesn't it? --"Good evening, Stella, oh Goddess of Feelgood, will you bless me with a joint?")

The first recorded use of cannabis therapeutically was in the 28th Century BC in China. The emperor, Shen-Nung, since he was the supreme being at the time, decided that he was a doctor. He prescribed cannabis for beriberi, constipation, "female weakness," gout, malaria, rheumatism and absentmindedness. This was a great medical breakthrough as all of the patients assured the emperor they had become completely well -- a 100 percent cure rate. (It beat moxibustion, the red-hot iron or a hole bored in the head.) In the second Century BC, pot was used for the treatment of appendicitis. In retrospect, it was a good way to make the diagnosis. If you didn't have appendicitis, you got well. If you did have appendicitis, you died.

The current argument about whether we should use marijuana medically or, in the eyes of some, even test it medically, seems ludicrous when studying the recent history of the weed. In the age of Napoleon, cannabis became widely accepted by Western medical practitioners. Between 1840 and 1890, more than 100 articles were published recommending pot for one disorder or another. As happens in medicine today, most of this was fad-driven, junk science. By 1937, cannabis had lost its image. It went from being a medicine to being a disreputable intoxicant, an image it richly deserved under the circumstances, and so it was outlawed nationwide in 1937. Now it is under investigation again as a medicine. Useful medicine or destroyer of souls? -- apparently, the American people can't let it be both at the same time. I'll have much more to say about marijuana, in a medical context, later.

Another addictive smoking substance, getting a bad press lately, is tobacco. Yet, when it was first introduced in Europe, it was described as a health-giving herb. And recent science indicates that, within reason (like everything else), this is true. Tobacco, presumably from the nicotine, is effective in treating the mental lassitude of Alzheimer's disease. See my book, The Smoker's Paradox -- The Health Benefits of Tobacco -- (order from Rhino Publishing's Website: www.rhinopublish.com or request an order form at 416-352-5126)

We're by no means the first society to become hysterical, to the point of self-enslavement, over drugs. Coffee was introduced into the middle east in 1510. The Mullahs said it was forbidden in the Koran (even though the Koran was written long before coffee came along.) What were the great centers of sin and sedition? -- coffeehouses! When the Mullahs realized that the people weren't buying the line that Allah doesn't drink coffee, and their reign of terror was having no effect whatsoever, the coffeehouses were reopened.

Pliny, another of the respected physicians of antiquity, had definite ideas about which types of pain were the worst. He said: "...to try to distinguish which ailment is the most terrible seems almost like folly as each believes his present ill to be the most cruel of all." But then he nominated, from his experience, what he considered to be nature's worst tormentors: "On this point, however, experience has shown that the disorders that cause the most atrocious torments are stones in the urethra while pains in the stomach are in second place, and headaches in third; there are few other complaints that lead to suicide." (Pliny, *Natural History*, Book XXV)

And bleeding was recognized as a potent pain reliever, even into the 19th Century. In the 1790s, Philip Syng Physick of Philadelphia, the father of American surgery, bled a patient into a state of collapse before manipulating a dislocated joint. He reported that the patient was entirely relaxed and seemed insensitive to pain. The patient was "relaxed" because he was in hemorrhagic shock and near death. Bloodletting was also used to "ease births" in the early 19th century. Is it any wonder that often the baby would live but the mother would die? Doctors have always been dangerous ("Bumper stickers" were different in horse-and-buggy days. The most popular one, seen on the tailgate or the rump of almost every horse, declared: "Guns

Don't Kill People -- Doctors Do") so perhaps it's not as bad as it used to be.

In the Middle Ages, there was an ambivalence about pain. The doctors and the priesthood were, in a sense, in competition for the management of pain. While the doctors would attempt to alleviate pain, although in ways that sometimes seem irrational to us, the priesthood saw pain as a divine retribution or as a sign that the sufferer had been especially chosen and would thus get rewards in the hereafter. But, although the Church tried to get its flock to accept pain as something to be endured as a "divine gift" or a sacrifice that brought them closer to God, there is no evidence that men and women were any tougher in enduring pain than they are today. Many preferred to wait for death rather than endure a tearing or burning of the flesh. There were exceptions, of course, such as the previously-mentioned Napoleonic horsemen in the Russian war who would have a limb amputated and, in a few days, mount up and go back into battle. (That is so remarkable that I thought it worth mentioning again.)

Michel de Montaigne, a 16th Century philosopher, who is little known and thus little read, had this to say about pain: "Thus, let us concern ourselves only with pain which, I grant you willingly, is the worst misfortune to befall us and, of any man in the world, I am certainly the one to wish it the identical ill and to do my utmost to avoid it so that, up to the present, I have not had, thanks be to God, much to do with it. But it is in us, if not to eradicate it, at least to decrease it by perseverance; but should the body yet be affected by it, nevertheless it is necessary to keep the soul and mind steadfast." Later in life, he suffered greatly and had "much to do with it."

Some men seem to be talented in almost every direction. Sir Christopher Wren, like Michelangelo, was one of these men. Wren designed St. Paul's Cathedral in London. He was a professor of astronomy at Oxford University and an enthusiastic scientist, making his mark even in the field of medicine. In fact, Wren is credited with administering the first successful intravenous anesthetic in 1659.

To satisfy his curiosity about both opium and alcohol, Wren injected a dog with opium in warm sack (sherry). The dog was totally anesthetized and recovered with no untoward effects. But the doctors didn't get it and it was another 200 years before intravenous anesthesia caught on.

Also in the 16th century, Valerius Cordus synthesized ether and called his compound "sweet vitriol." Cordus did not realize the importance of his discovery and so missed his chance at medical mortality. Paracelsus, a contemporary of Cordus, noted sweet vitriol's sleep-inducing properties and remarked that it "quiets all suffering without any harm and relieves all pain, and quenches all fevers, and prevents complications in all disease." Despite the rave reviews by one of the top doctors of the time, Paracelsus, the healing powers of "sweet vitriol," entered the 18th Century unnoticed as an anesthetic. Ether was <u>rediscovered</u> by Michael Faraday somewhat later (see below).

In the 18th Century, the antipodes of medical pain treatment vs. the Church's attitude regarding pain continued. Was pain an evil to be vanquished by the physician or was it God's punishment for original sin? Christian theology implies that God is good, forgiving and omnipotent. So, does God want his creatures to suffer? What about innocent children and animals who can hardly be guilty of original sin? No matter what the opinions of the Church in this period, doctors and patients sought relief from pain -- and left the philosophy to the Church.

In the previous Century, Pascal went along with the Church rather than science, such as it was. He proclaimed: "Whatever discretions the Church used, it was always clear that if it were accepted that Man's ultimate purpose on earth was to both serve and love God, then health was no more important in itself than any other earthly possession. It also followed that illness and pain could be viewed as benefits." I doubt that Pascal had a booming practice since the only reason people went to a doctor was for relief of pain.

Hippocrates, the Father of Medicine and the last word on a lot of things, did not agree with

Pascal and stated many centuries before him: "One could in general say that since nothing which causes pain is beneficial, it must always be regarded as detrimental in its own right, be it alone, or linked to another illness, because it depletes strength, upsets the functions, it stops the digestion of 'morbific' humors, (and) depending on its intensity, it always produces some of the detrimental effects mentioned above."

Hippocrates, as usual, was thousands of years ahead of his time. Modern science has "discovered" that severe pain <u>depresses healing</u>."...it always produces," said the good Doctor Hippocrates, "some of the detrimental effects mentioned above."

Opium, or some form of opiate, has been in man's kitchen or bathroom cabinet for over 4,000 years. After the passage of four millennia, there is little new in the field. It seems odd that, after all this history on the use of these God-given forms of pain relief, many doctors are uncertain, ignorant or fearful of their use.

In the 11th century, Avicenna referred to opium as "the most powerful of stupefacients." It was freely used in Western medicine from the 16th to the 20th centuries, <u>often in massive doses</u>. Today, the opium derivatives--morphine, heroin, and codeine, in addition to cocaine -- continue to hold the key to pain relief but, unfortunately, the government now holds that key and they have made their usual mess of things.

THE MAGICAL GASES -- FOR SOIRÉE AND SURGERY

In 1772, Joseph Priestley identified nitrous oxide, the first gas recognized to have anesthetic powers. More than 20 years later, when Humphry Davy experimented with inhaling nitrous oxide, he was taken by the distinctly pleasant results. He felt giddy, his muscles relaxed, and his hearing seemed more acute. Because the compound made him want to laugh, he dubbed it "laughing gas." About two decades later, Davy's student Michael Faraday studied the pain-relieving effects of sulfuric ether and compared them with those of nitrous oxide.

In 1824, Henry Hill Hickman, a contemporary of Faraday and Davy, carried out painless operations on animals using carbon dioxide anesthesia to create a condition he called "suspended animation." Although he failed to arouse much interest, Hickman managed to win the approval of Baron Dominique-Jean Larrey, the most famous surgeon of Napoleon's day.

Following Dr. Hickman's lead, Dr. Larrey also espoused carbon dioxide anesthesia to induce "suspended animation." This would be considered outrageous today, as CO2 can kill, but perhaps doctors of the time had forgotten about opium. If Dr. Larrey was amputating your leg at the hip joint, would you have risked asphyxiation from CO_2 or gone cold turkey? (I think I know your answer.)

"Both ether and nitrous oxide were well known in the first half of the 19th century. Physicians in the United States used ether to treat pulmonary tuberculosis, while the general public was often drawn to lectures by itinerant professors expounding on the mysteries and magic of gases. These lectures often included demonstrations in which volunteers from the audience were given doses of ether or nitrous oxide. This usually brought on a state of drunkenness and hilarity." (O'Brien, M.E., *Relief of Suffering: Where the Art and Science of Medicine Meet.* Postgraduate Medicine, 1996;99(6):189-208).

The person commonly regarded as the discoverer of anesthesia was a Boston dentist, William T. G. Morton. On September 20, 1846, Morton used ether for extraction of a tooth from one of his patients. Thereafter, anesthesia was quickly accepted. Medical opposition was virtually nonexistent--except for childbirth. Amazingly, no fatalities were reported during these early years. But even if the risks had been appreciated, freedom from pain superseded the fear of death.

Chloroform was discovered virtually simultaneously in 1831 by doctors in the US, Germany and France (a common occurrence in science). However, it took 15 years for the medical profession to catch on to its utility in surgery.

An English obstetrician, Dr. James Young Simpson, became interested in chloroform. After trying it on himself and <u>guests at a dinner party</u> -- a popular experimental group in the 19th Century -- Simpson introduced it into his obstetric practice.

Priests and ministers objected to this evil practice, saying that "God intended birth to be painful." The pious public considered it immoral to reduce women to a state of unconsciousness at the moment of creation, so to speak. When rumors spread that anesthetics brought on erotic fantasies, transforming birth into an imagined orgasm, fears multiplied. (Having the comparable experience of <u>passing a baby elephant</u>, or having an "Imagined orgasm," which do you suppose the mothers chose?)

Queen Victoria took chloroform for the birth of her eighth child, Prince Leopold, in 1853 and had the "imagined orgasm" again for the birth of Princess Beatrice, four years later. John Snow, history's first anesthesiologist, did the honors in both births -- and that was the end of resistance to obstetic anesthesia. Parenthetically, Victoria also used marijuana for her headaches. Today she would have to be imprisoned or at least forced into some sort of treatment program.

****

Aspirin has been around, in one form or another, since 1830. But it was 70 years before it was recognized as a pain reliever.

The narcotic powers of the coca plant had been known in the West since the 16th century, but it remained unused as a narcotic for 150 years. Through the efforts of Sigmund Freud and Dr. Carl Koller, an ophthalmologist, cocaine became immensely popular after 1884. It remained universally accepted as a boon for suffering patients until the Great Drug War of the late 20th Century put cocaine out on the street instead of in the doctor's office.

Just a year after Koller's demonstration of the efficacy of cocaine in ophthalmology, William Halsted established neuroregional anesthesia using cocaine. He reported success with more than 1,000 surgical cases. Halsted became "addicted" to cocaine and routinely used it (or morphine) during his years as top surgeon in the United States.

Attempts to synthesize the anesthetic agent in cocaine were successful in about 1900. Procaine ("Novocain"), after 50 years, is still the most popular local anesthetic world-wide.

THE MIDDLE 19TH CENTURY -- A REGRESSION TO NAPOLEONIC METHODS OF PAIN CONTROL: FOUR STOUT MEN, A BOTTLE OF WHISKEY AND A RAG TO CHEW ON

Our War Between the States is a sad example of a missed opportunity to avoid much of the horror of war injuries. The marvelous anesthetic effect of chloroform had been known for exactly <u>30 years</u> and was being widely used in Europe. In fact, one of the co-discoverers of chloroform was an American.

Anesthesia caught hold quickly soon thereafter, but too late for the millions who suffered in that Great American Holocaust.

General anesthesia was so dramatic! One moment the patient is awake and jabbering or crying, and the next he's like a sleeping baby -- what doctor could resist it? Try suturing a laceration on a screaming two-year-old and you will see what I mean. (When I was faced with this ordeal, I used to go out of sight, stuff cotton in my ears and reappear with a benign smile on my face. For some strange reason, many of the nurses thought this was a callous thing to do. I just don't understand women.)

Analgesic agents took much longer to be accepted. Aspirin was king for the first half of the 20th century until acetaminophen was introduced in 1955. I'm still holding out for aspirin. I think it is a better analgesic than Tylenol. However, Tylenol is better than Darvon, which came along in the 60s, is worthless and addicting to boot.

---

* The northern side had some general anesthetic -- chloroform and ether -- but the south had to get by with whiskey, brute strength and the rag in the mouth.

The ibuprofen agents became available by prescription-only in the 1970s; they hit the over-the-counter market in 1984. There are now dozens of nonsteroidal anti-inflammatory drugs [NSAIDs] available both by prescription and over-the-counter. Why are some of them over-the-counter and others by prescription only? I think it's because they want the doctor to do the experimenting on you with the new variety of drug. If it turns out to kill you or maim you for life, you can sue the doctor. You wouldn't get very far suing the druggist. (Remember, bureaucrats envy and hate doctors.) I think the NSAIDS are also over rated for pain relief. However, there is such a powerful placebo effect in treating mild-to-moderate pain that no one knows for sure.

The techniques for pain relief have become increasingly sophisticated, the administration of drugs has been infinitely refined, and pain-relieving drugs have proliferated. Though the application of these pain relievers has been, ironically, less than enthusiastic.

There are now many dozens of "pain-killers" in pill form on the market. What does that tell you? It means there's probably not much difference between them and it's all based on personal prejudice (like mine for aspirin). If you study the ingredients on a dozen boxes of pain medicine, you will see there is little difference between them.

"Many health professionals," says Dr. Mary E. O'Brien, "are now taking a fresh look at some old pain-relieving techniques. Non-drug measures, such as massage, aromatherapy, prayer, yoga meditation, guided imagery, relaxation, music, and laughter, are being incorporated in pain management programs. The mind-body connection, ignored for centuries, has been reestablished."

I have not been impressed with these alternative methods for pain relief except in mild-to-moderate cases. The most effective of these alternatives, not mentioned by Dr. O'Brien, is acupuncture.

Dr. O'Brien supports the current trend toward allowing patients in severe pain, especially in the hospital setting, to control their own medication. And "...a goal for the future is to prevent pain before it starts." That's an ambitious project and one worth pursuing. A pre-surgical plan for an operation that is certain to elicit pain at a certain region, abdominal pain after abdominal surgery as an example, is an innovative and possibly rewarding field of pain research.

Why not, for instance, try color therapy over the operated area before and following knee surgery? Preposterous? Well, maybe. But what harm would it do to have an orthopedist, who is not worried about his image, illuminate the surgical wound with blue light for a few days pre- and post-surgical? Wouldn't it be wonderful if it turned out to dramatically decrease post-surgical pain and also accelerated the healing process? Sometimes simple and effective remedies are ignored for centuries. See my book,

COLOR ME HEALTHY -- Order from Rhino Publishing's Website: www.rhinopublish.com or request an order form at 416-352-5126.

I feel certain that a presurgical sphenopalatine ganglion block, using liquid cocaine [explained elsewhere in this book], would relieve an enormous amount of post-surgical pain. The insane War on Drugs has made cocaine available only to addicts and criminals but not to the suffering patient. More on this criminal collusion between the executive branch of the federal government, local police and the underworld later on.

Dr. O'Brien concluded: "As our population ages, we are being faced with increasingly complex questions about how to help patients who will not get better." The future of pain relief depends on rethinking some old attitudes about the nature of pain. Like the father who didn't want his dying son to receive morphine because the boy might become addicted, physicians need to take a hard look at the value of narcotics and the possibility that inadequate treatment will only make a bad situation worse.

"As our nation and profession chart a course for the next several decades, pain probably won't top the list of medical priorities," she added sadly.

Our society has made tremendous strides in saving and extending lives, but with the federal takeover of medicine, there has been a serious deterioration in the humanity of medicine and poor or no treatment of pain is a prime example of this deterioration. Pain matters, at least to patients, and they will increasingly make their needs known. At least there is now enough awareness of the neglect and hypocrisy that has been extant in this important field of medicine, that there is real hope for change.

The remarkable thing to me is that the medical profession, including the nurses, have been so callous about pain over the past half Century. In 1941, I had a football "back" injury that turned out to be a severe kidney contusion. I had to have numerous cystoscopies (insertion of a cystoscopic tube through the penis), which was pretty tough on a 15-year-old kid.

But back then, there was no question about completely relieving post-surgical pain. I was given Demerol adequate to make me perfectly comfortable. To say I was comfortable is an understatement. The mental and emotional state was comparable to a continual orgasm with tranquility thrown in. I didn't care if the hospital burned down right around me. But did I become addicted? Did I crave more? I left the hospital and never thought about it again until years later. When I do think about it now, it is when I see a child suffering unnecessary pain.

Throughout history, pain and medicine have gone hand-in-hand. This is obviously a truism but attitudes toward pain change with the times, not only the doctor's attitude but that of the patient. The flagellants of the Middle ages, for instance, tormented themselves in ways that seem preposterous today. They would not only inflict blows upon themselves but apply red-hot coals and branding irons to their bodies. Napoleon's soldiers, during the Russian campaign, would have a limb amputated and then go back into battle on horseback. In the Good Old Days in India, if you were lucky, you could have yourself pierced through the abdomen and hung to swing on a hook. By doing this, you were contributing to an abundant harvest and increasing the fertility of the people.

From these jolly times we have inherited the expression, "getting off the hook." Pain is not so hard to endure when it is being inflicted upon someone else, especially if it is helping the crops. and promoting fecundity.

During much of the history of medicine, pain has been considered a necessary part of the healing process, -- laudable pain, so to speak. In ancient Greece, if you were a criminal, the odds were you would not die an easy death. You would get lots of pain -- and it would not be laudable. Anatomists Herophilus and Erasistratus were given live criminals by the king from the dungeons for dissection "so they might capture in the raw what nature had kept hidden from them..." (The History of Pain, Rey, Harvard University Press, 1999)

Some physicians in "the age of enlightenment" believed in "laudable pain" to the extent that they would inflict pain in order to cure it! They would use cautery, friction, flagellation and urtication. These various forms of torture "would provoke a beneficial discharge and awakening sensibility." One of the most popular methods to fight pain with pain was "moxibustion," which consisted of a stiff fabric "stick" with vegetable fibers in it. This burning concoction was placed on the skin "to create a diversionary point."

Aretaeus of Cappadocia, who lived in Rome in 100, AD, was an exceptionally fine physician in that his descriptions of diseases were remarkably accurate and still apply to this day. But on the treatment side he was a victim of his times, having little to work with. For migraine headache, for instance, he would first do bloodletting of the arm and then the forehead. Then the head was shaved and hot towels were applied to prepare the shaved head for scarification and cupping (more blood loss). Then to stop the bleeding, a branding iron was applied to the head wounds. (I wonder how many Florents they paid for that stimulating therapy.) When all this failed, the old reliable trephination was used. There's nothing like a hole in the head, according to the experts of the time, to relieve your headache. The ancient Egyptians had invented this clever therapy thousands of years earlier.

Speaking of the popular branding iron, a famous surgeon, Hermann Boerhaave, who had a disease syndrome named after him, was in favor of the frequent use of the red-hot iron, especially in cases of hysteria and convulsions, which, apparently, he considered to be psychological. He was convinced that just the threat of the branding iron "would be enough to suppress all such symptoms of disorder" --and I'll bet it worked.

Dioscorides, who lived in the time of Aretaeus mentioned above, was very familiar with narcotics 1900 years ago. One gets the impression, from reading the history of those times that, like today, narcotics were not used as extensively as they should have been. Among the pain-killers available were the opium poppy, the field poppy, marijuana, alcohol, lettuce, belladonna, henbane and black nightshade.

Marijuana, you may be surprised to learn, has been used in medicine for <u>five thousand years</u>. Marijuana is mentioned five times in the Bible under such names as kaneh or kannabus which is translated into "aromatic cane" or "sweet cane." The first three mentions in the Bible (Exodus 30:22-23; Song of Songs 4:4-14; Isaiah 43:23-24) are highly favorable to its use. The last two (Jeremiah 6:20; Ezekiel 27:19) are neutral if not negative. Yahweh's adherents favored cannabis, another name for marijuana, as did the worshipers of the Hebrew god, Ashteroth or Astarte, known as "Queen of Heaven," "Star of the Sea," and "Stella Maris." (Now that sounds like a pot-smoking goddess, doesn't it? -- "Good evening, Stella, oh Goddess of Feelgood, will you bless me with a joint?")

The first recorded use of cannabis therapeutically was in the 28th Century BC in China. The emperor, Shen-Nung, since he was the supreme being at the time, decided that he was a doctor. He prescribed cannabis for beriberi, constipation, "female weakness," gout, malaria, rheumatism and absentmindedness. This was a great medical breakthrough as all of the patients assured the emperor they had become completely well -- a 100 percent cure rate. (It beat moxibustion, the red hot iron or a hole bored in the head.) In the second Century BC, pot was used for the treatment of appendicitis. In retrospect, it was a good way to make the diagnosis. If you didn't have appendicitis, you got well. If you did have appendicitis, you died.

The current argument about whether we should use marijuana medically or, in the eyes of some, even test it medically, seems ludicrous when studying the recent history of the weed. In the age of Napoleon, cannabis became widely accepted by Western medical practitioners. Between 1840 and 1890, more than 100 articles were published recommending pot for one disorder or another. As happens in medicine today, most of this was fad-driven, junk science. By 1937, cannabis had lost its image. It went from being a medicine to being a disreputable intoxicant, an image it richly deserved under the circumstances, and so it was outlawed nationwide in 1937 Now it is under investigation again as a medicine. Useful medicine or destroyer of souls? -- apparently, the American people can't let it be both at the same time. I'll have much more to say about marijuana, in a medical context, later.

Another addictive smoking substance, getting a bad press lately, is tobacco. Yet, when it was first introduced in Europe, it was described as a health-giving herb. And recent science indicates that, within reason (like everything else), this is true. Tobacco, presumably from the nicotine, is effective in treating the mental lassitude of Alzheimer's disease.

We're by no means the first society to become hysterical, to the point of self-enslavement, over drugs. Coffee was introduced into the middle east in 1510. The Mullahs said it was forbidden in the Koran (even though the Koran was written long before coffee came along.) What were the great centers of sin and sedition? -- coffeehouses! When the Mullahs realized that the people weren't buying the line that Allah doesn't drink coffee, and their reign of terror was having no effect whatsoever, the coffeehouses were reopened.

Pliny, another of the respected physicians of antiquity, had definite ideas about which types of pain were the worst. He said: "...to try to distinguish which ailment is the most terrible seems almost like folly as each believes his present ill to be the most cruel of all." But then he nominated, from his experience, what he considered to be nature's worst tormentors: "On this point, however, experience has shown that the disorders that cause the most atrocious torments are stones in the urethra while pains in the stomach are in second place, and headaches in third; there are few other complaints that lead to suicide." (Pliny, *Natural History*, Book XXV)

In the Middle Ages, there was an ambivalence about pain. The doctors and the priesthood were, in a sense, in competition for the managemant of pain. While the doctors would attempt to alleviate pain, although in ways that sometimes seem irrational to us, the priesthood saw pain as a divine retribution or as a sign that the sufferer had been especially chosen and would thus get rewards in the hereafter. But, although the Church tried to get its flock to accept pain as something to be endured as a "divine gift" or a sacrifice that brought them closer to God, there is no evidence that men and women were any tougher in enduring pain than they are today. Many preferred to wait for death rather than endure a tearing or burning of the flesh. There were exceptions, of course, such as the previously-mentioned Napoleonic horsemen in the Russian war who would have a limb amputated and, in a few days, mount up and go back into battle. (That is so remarkable that I thought it worth mentioning again.)

Michel de Montaigne, a 16th Century philosopher, who is little known and thus little read, had this to say about pain: "Thus, let us concern ourselves only with pain which, I grant you willingly, is the worst misfortune to befall us and, of any man in the world, I am certainly the one to wish it the identical ill and to do my utmost to avoid it so that, up to the present, I have not had, thanks be to God, much to do with it. But it is in us, if not to eradicate it, at least to decrease it by perseverance; but should the body yet be affected by it, nevertheless it is necessary to keep the soul and mind steadfast." Later in life, he suffered greatly and had "much to do with it."

In the 18th Century, the antipodes of medical pain treatment vs. the Church's attitude regarding pain continued. Was pain an evil to be vanquished by the physician or was it God's punishment for original sin? Christian theology implies that God is good, forgiving and omnipotent. So, does God want his creatures to suffer? What about innocent children and animals who can hardly be guilty of original sin? No matter what the opinions of the Church in this period, doctors and patients sought relief from pain -- and left the philosophy to the Church.

In the previous Century, Pascal went along with the Church rather than science, such as it was. He proclaimed: "Whatever discretions the Church used, it was always clear that if it were accepted that Man's ultimate purpose on earth was to both serve and love God, then health was no more important in itself than any other earthly possession. It also followed that illness and pain could be viewed as benefits." I doubt that Pascal had a booming practice since the only reason people went to a doctor was for relief of pain.

Hippocrates, the Father of Medicine and the last word on a lot of things, did not agree with Pascal and stated many centuries before him: "One could in general say that since nothing which causes pain is beneficial, it must always be regarded as detrimental in its own right, be it alone, or linked to another illness, because it depletes strength, upsets the functions, it stops the digestion of 'morbific' humors, (and) depending on its intensity, it always produces some of the detrimental effects mentioned above."

Hippocrates, as usual, was thousands of years ahead of his time. Modern science has "discovered" that severe pain depresses healing. "...it always produces," said the good Doctor Hippocrates, "some of the detrimental effects mentioned above."

There is an interesting lesson that we should have learned from the introduction of heroin. It was introduced as a non-addicting pain reliever, the perfect non-addicting substitute for morphine! Heroin, diacetylmorphine, was synthesized in 1874. By the turn of the Century, it was being peddled all over the world by the German Bayer company along with aspirin, often in the same ad. German scientists tested it and concluded that heroin was an excellent therapy for bronchitis (which it is) chronic coughing and asthma (which it is) and tuberculosis (which it isn't.) Free samples of heroin were sent out to physicians for distribution to their patients and, in 1906, the American Medical Association approved herion for general use and recommended that it be used as a non-addicting substitute for morphine "in various painful conditions." Keep in mind that heroin is five times as potent as morphine.

Naturally, the above-described flight into therapeutic madness led to a huge addiction problem for the unsuspecting public as well as addicts who wanted their drugs as high octane as possible -- 200,000 addicts by 1924, the year it was finally outlawed.

This incredible bungle brings to mind a question: If the pharmaceutical industry and the AMA were that short-sighted and incompetent in 1924, what about now? Are they really competent enough to judge whether you need pain relief or not? Shouldn't you be the judge of that, or would you rather be treated like a child and assume the doctor knows best?

Parenthetically, the percentage of hard core addicts hasn't changed in the last 75 years. So what has the war on drugs accomplished? The only thing it has accomplished is the turning of America into a police state.

Cocaine has a similar history to heroin in that everyone trusted industry and medicine and thought cocaine was harmless. It was added to Coca-Cola until 1903, hence the "Coca" in Coca-Cola. It was available for snorting as a treatment for sinusitis and hay fever. Sigmund Freud enthusiastically recommended it for depression and the American company, Parke-Davis, not to be out done by Germany's Bayer, sold it in many forms for drinking, smoking or rubbing on the skin.

"LAUDABLE PAIN"

It was commonly believed by doctors of the 19th Century that pus in the wound of an operation was essential, or at least contributory to, healing. It was called "laudable pus." Perhaps even more remarkable was the belief that pain was a necessary element in the healing process --"laudable pain," so to speak. However, the best doctors of the time did not hold with this heartless belief of the medical majority.

Dominique-Jean Larrey, the greatest surgeon of the 19th Century who served Napoleon through all of his campaigns, from Austerlitz to

Waterloo to Egypt, was a strong exponent of giving patients as much pain relief as possible. He clearly understood that pain was the enemy of the patient, not a friend. The American surgeon, Dr. Agnew was a great admirer of Larrey: "As an operator, he was judicious but bold and rapid; calm and self-possessed in every emergency; but full of feeling and tenderness. He stands among the military surgeons where Napoleon stands among the generals, the first and the greatest."

Larrey was criticized by some of his surgical competitors for his quickness to amputate. Faure, for example, said: "...there is more honor in saving a limb than in amputating it with dexterity and success."

Larrey explained his reasons for quick action: the benefits of the early state of shock brought on by massive wounds -- patients often, in fact usually, do not remember the first few hours following the trauma. To delay was to invite infection, prolonged suffering and death. In those days of rampant gangrene and the horror of surgery without anesthesia, Larrey was, in my opinion, the better doctor.

Ref: *Surgical Memoirs of Campaigns*, Philadelphia, 1832
The Catholic Encyclopedia, Vol. IX

1. Wall PD, Jones M. Defeating pain: the war against a silent epidemic. New York: Plenum, 1991

2. O'Brien ME. Relief of suffering: where the art and science of medicine meet. Postgraduate Medicine, 1996;99(6):189-208

3. White PF. Use of patient-controlled analgesia for management of acute pain. Journal of the American Medical Association, 1988;259(2):243-7

4. Solomon S. Overcoming barriers to effective pain management. Postgraduate Medicine: A Special Report, Oct 1996

5. Gorman C. The case for morphine. Time 1997 Apr 28:64-5

6 Postgraduate Medicine, July, 1997, Mary E. O'Brien, MD

7. The History of Pain, Roselyne Rey, Harvard University Press, 1995

****

DOCTORS AND PAIN

An expert on pain recently stated in an article in Scientific American: "As common as it is, pain can be extremely elusive. The patient may have difficulty describing it, and the physician often cannot substantiate it. An individual in acute pain may scream and writhe in agony; but the person with chronic pain often appears outwardly normal, with few visible signs. This makes it difficult for the doctor and the patient."

If the doctor cannot substantiate the pain by palpation of the affected part or by X-ray or other "scientific" means, he immediately becomes suspicious and defensive: Is this patient just looking for attention? Is he an addict? Is he crazy?

I know all about these mental mechanisms. As a young doctor, I reacted the same way. And that was long before the present drug paranoia when you could prescribe all the narcotic you felt the patient needed with no questions asked. Those were indeed the Good Old Days from the patient's point of view, at least to a point. But we were all afflicted with the fear of addiction, drug tolerance and respiratory depression and so, although better than today's paralysis in the field of pain relief, it was less than perfect and many patients suffered terribly because of our ignorance and unfounded fears of addiction.

Pain is difficult for the patient to describe and the physician to evaluate. Although much remains to be learned about the mechanism of pain, we know individuals have different levels of tolerance to pain. There are also differences in individual sensitivity to drugs, and in how drugs are metabolized. Studies indicate that pain relief from opiates varies by age, race, cultural differences, type of pain and location of pain. Because the effectiveness of pain medication varies greatly from person to person, <u>a patient's need for a high dose is not necessarily a sign of addiction</u>.

With the same affliction, some people hurt more than others. It will not do to consider them weak, childish or stupid just because they experience more pain than what you think is "proper" for that illness. As a young doctor, I didn't understand this; pain was pain and that's all there was to it. It seemed obvious, even to my young brain, that all pains were not equal but I thought each type of pain should be more or less the same in each person. You learn otherwise after you have experienced a little pain yourself. Maybe no one under the age of 50 should be allowed to take care of pain patients. A little personal experience in the field of pain is a great teacher.

Which experiences pain the most, men or women? Many studies suggest that women report or feel pain more acutely than men, and are more likely to report to a pain center for treatment. However, it's not clear if the difference is due to women actually experiencing more pain, or sociologic, with men less likely to admit they are having a problem -- the old stiff-upper-lip attitude.

Studies have shown that women perceive taste sensations, such as sweet, sour, bitter or salty, at lower levels of concentration than men, i.e., they are more sensitive to these stimuli. They can more easily detect an electrical stimulus as well. This difference is heightened during the luteal phase of menstruation, the time just after ovulation. While studies on pain perception have had conflicting results, laboratory research suggests that women do also have a lower tolerance to pain or, put another way, are more sensitive to pain. Some studies have shown that if women are supplemented with oral contraceptives during the luteal phase of the menstrual cycle, the threshold for pain is the same as for males. This isn't absolutely proven, this relationship of hormones to pain sensitivity, because the studies were small.

And the smell sensitivity of women, in my experience, is quite remarkable compared to men. They must have olfactory nerves twice the size of ours. During a period when I was experiencing bad breath from an undetected abscessed tooth, my daughter could detect that I hadn't cleaned my teeth from <u>across the room</u> -- "Daddy, you've been eating sheep dung again!" Enough about women and on to children.

Dr. F. Michael Ferrante, director of the Anesthesia Pain Management Program at the University of Pennsylvania School of Medicine in Philadelphia, says that children and infants experience pain exactly as adults. If you don't think so, watch a newborn baby having a circumcision immediately after birth — it's really barbaric to welcome a baby into the world with such torture. One pain expert has remarked: "...it can be difficult to determine the extent of pain that newborns experience." Well I guess he's never witnessed a circumcision.

Pain in and of itself can be hazardous, whether or not an infant remembers the sensation. Pain increases the heart rate, blood pressure and stress hormones, and a 1992 study found that babies undergoing surgery had less morbidity, mortality, and complications if they were given a deep anesthetic compared to light sedation. Some people just don't seem to think babies are human (in or out of the womb.) If you are going to have your little guy circumcised -- and I do not recommend it -- make the doctor promise to use a local anesthetic.

How would you like to come into this world and, within an hour, be faced with <u>surgery without anesthesia</u>? If you are a male, there is a good chance that is exactly what happened to you in the form of circumcision -- no wonder you are so neurotic about pain.

The theory was that even if the infants felt the pain, they would not remember it. They feel it, I can assure you. I did my share of circumcisions as a medical student and intern and I always felt queasy about it. The poor little guys screamed bloody murder. The residents would always assure me that it was all right, as they didn't remember it. I was just an ignorant student -- what did I know? But what did <u>HE</u> know? Not much, it seems, because research has shown with rats that the body <u>does</u> remember the pain.

For years, doctors operated on premature babies without anesthesia in the belief that even if the infants felt the pain, they would not remember it. New research with rats suggests that the body does remember the pain <u>and is forever changed</u>. Using newborn rats, researchers at the National Institutes of Health found that painful trauma that mimics medical procedures commonly performed on premature infants caused the rats to become much more sensitive to pain as they grew older.

M. A. Ruda, a NIH researcher, opines that the reason for this "pain remembered" is that pain causes the developing nervous system of the very young to grow more nerve cells that carry the sensation of pain to the brain.

"We found that there are more nerve endings that fire and transmit the (pain) information," said Ruda. "These animals later were more sensitive and had a greater response to pain."

Animal studies of pain have been consistently valid for predicting the responses that one sees in humans.

The study is part of a continuing effort by medical science to understand how and when the nervous system develops and how the growth of nerve tissue is affected by stimulation, such as pain.

Such research has a direct bearing on efforts to save and improve the lives of infants born prematurely, before the normal 40-week gestation.

Survival of babies born up to 15 weeks premature is now not unusual, but it takes a major medical effort and many painful procedures, including countless needle sticks, breathing tubes and even surgery to save these tiny ones.

"Just how much pain such babies feel has been uncertain," said Dr. Patricia A. McGrath, a pain researcher and professor of pediatrics at the University of Western Ontario.

Uncertain? I don't know how you can make such a statement, Patricia. Haven't you ever carved on the penis of a newborn? You'd have to be blind, deaf and dumb not to see the agonizing pain these little guys go through. It's absolutely barbaric.

Ten years ago, she said, ``there was a real belief that the pain system in premature babies was not developed and these infants would really not feel as much pain." Well, there are a lot of blind, deaf and dumb doctors in this world.

Microscopic examination of nerves in injured animals shows why they experience more pain than uninjured ones. Nerves leading from an injured paw are much more dense than are the nerves in an untreated paw or in control animals. The increased density means there are more nerve circuits to carry pain stimuli to the brain.

Ruda said other studies have shown that premature babies tend to report more pain in their childhood years and their parents report that these children's pain response is greater than in their siblings.

"We use anesthesia as well as we can in these babies," Dr. Jonelle C. Rowe, an NIH doctor said. "A major research effort is under way to find the best way to safely relieve medical-procedure pain in the very young."

It has been a long time in coming. It's a shame they have neglected the field of *pain in the very young* because of this myth that babies don't experience the same degree of pain as "humans." [When <u>do</u> they become human? I thought it was at <u>conception</u>. I'm a little old fashioned on this embryological concept. Seems to me they've changed the rules.

Ref: Associated Press, Paul Recer, 07/27/00

As I was writing this report, another pain study was reported in the lay press. The headline of the article gave the gist of the depressing story:

Hospitals Failing Post-op Pain Relief

"Many hospitals are not doing enough to control pain in surgical patients, according to a study of cases in hospitals in New York State," Reuters News reported. Dr. Charles Stimler, clinical coordinator with IPRO, a nonprofit health care quality improvement organization based in Albany, New York, said: "When it comes to reducing pain among surgical patients, there is considerable room for improvement" The organization studied 105 New York State hospitals. The researchers reviewed the preoperative, surgical, and postoperative pain management of 220 patients admitted to those hospitals for either knee or hip replacement surgeries.

If you have ever had a hip fracture or a severe knee injury, you know what pain is. The researchers discovered that the majority of patients did not receive pain relief as recommended in federal standards issued in 1992 by the Department of Health and Human Services' Agency for Health Care Policy Research (AHCPR).

Now I think it's a little weird when the government is mandating that doctors give pain relief from one agency and at the same time they are fighting doctors trying to give pain relief from a dozen other agencies but, for what it's worth, here's what the government "mandated": Eighty percent of each hospital's surgical patients (why not 100 percent?) should engage in preoperative discussions with hospital staff regarding their pain care. The IPRO survey, however, found that just 13% of the New York patients discussed such matters with care givers.

The AHCPR rules also mandate that 80% of all patients receive regular "pain evaluations" on the day of, as well as the day after, their surgery. Ideally, the agency says, these checks should occur every two hours. In reality, regular pain evaluations were carried out on the day of the operation in just 51% of cases studied by IPRO. This number fell to 45% for the day after surgery.

The AHCPR also advises <u>that hospitals offer 80% of patients the option of non-pharmaceutical, "alternative" pain relief techniques</u> such as biofeedback, relaxation therapies, acupuncture and hypnosis. However, according to the IPRO study, these alternative analgesic methods were only made available to 11% of patients. That lack of interest in alternatives will probably not surprise you.

Dr. Stimler said that patients must also become more active about voicing their concerns. "Patients need to ask the doctor or nurse what to expect, examine pain control options, and work with medical personnel to devise a suitable pain control plan." I hate to say this, but, if they seem uninterested in your concern about pain (you're just another sissy) then you might have to threaten them ("If you don't give me adequate pain relief I'm not going to donate that $ five million to the liver transplant unit.") <u>This is a last resort</u> and could be counterproductive. Maybe you could say it in a joking way. (Ref: Reuters News Service, Wed, 28 Oct, 1997)

****

If you want your doctor to know that you are really serious about pain relief, take your attorney with you to the surgeon's office, the day before the surgery. Introduce them and remark: "Mr. Swartz here is very concerned about my having proper pain relief and would like for you to sign this agreement, which states that you will give due consideration to my pain relief after surgery."

The best way to assure that you will have proper pain relief is to <u>hire a private nurse for the two nights following surgery</u>. The night shift is the period that your pain is most likely to be neglected. Ironically, as you know from your own illnesses, pain and discomfort always seems more intense at night. If you can afford it, it would be best to have a private nurse around the clock for the first 24 hours.

Many patients might not be aware that various pain management strategies even exist. For example, postoperative recovery can be accompanied with a regular schedule of pills or shots provided by staff; or it can be self-administered by the patient, so that when he presses a button, analgesia is automatically delivered through an intravenous line.

Finally, the experts said, no patient should worry about being a "bother" -- nursing staff are there to help. Letting care givers know about the extent of your discomfort is important -- persistent pain could be signaling a postoperative complication that requires attention.

PAIN THERAPY

A variety of methods are used to treat chronic pain. They may include acupuncture, biofeedback and other relaxation techniques, physical therapy, psychotherapy, hypnosis, chiropractic, behavior modification, nerve block by injection and transcutaneous electrical nerve stimulation (TENS). In addition, cancer patients who suffer pain may benefit from radiation therapy. This is usually due to shrinkage of a tumor mass compressing a nerve.

Surgery can alter the perception of pain, by modifying conduction of pain along pathways to the central nervous system, or as a last resort, block pain by cutting nerve bundles. Then again, this treatment may, paradoxically, make the pain worse or have no effect. The pain often can get to the brain even though the pathways to the brain have, supposedly, been severed. This is due to alternate pathways that are not understood. Needless to say, this was a disappointment and a surprise to surgeons. Medicine is not nuts and bolts; there is much to be learned. Non-steroidal anti-inflammatory agents, anti-depressants and anti convulsants are among the medications used, usually with little effect.

Speaking of "alternate pathways" to the brain to allow the brain to recognize that you are having pain, "the last gateway" is the sphenopalatine ganglion. This is like a railroad yard in a big city where all the tracks come together. It is located back of the hard palate, where your throat starts. All pain, from headache to gout in your big toe, must enter this portal. Numbing this area with liquid cocaine by inserting cocaine-soaked Q tips in the nose and back to the SP ganglion, is remarkably effective in relieving <u>any</u> type of pain. I used it with astounding results for ten years while practicing in Georgia. I gave it up when I started smelling the black cloud of tyranny closing in on me. (I am sure my daughter would have smelled it sooner.) I had a choice: stop helping these people or go to jail and never practice again.

Despite the variety of treatments available, a substantial number of pain patients are not helped. Even some of those successfully treated to a certain extent must learn to live with pain under the present governmental constraints.

Narcotics are extremely effective for pain relief, but their long term use has been avoided because of the irrational fear of addiction that we have discussed at length. Included are "opiates" like morphine and codeine, which are derived from opium, and "opioids" like heroin -- five times as powerful as morphine -- and methadone, which are synthetic or semisynthetic compounds with similar properties.

Opiate therapy is now generally used only for burn victims and terminal cancer patients, and, for shorter periods, for hospital patients

who have undergone surgery. The standard prescription is PRN which means "pro re nata", or
"as needed". In effect the order means medication is to be given only after pain returns. And
the nurse, who is not in pain, makes the decision if the patient is "really" in pain, or in
"enough" pain, or just "thinks" he is in pain.
However, by the time the pain is treated, it may
be so severe that a larger dose, with greater side
effects, is needed. The ideal treatment is to stay
ahead of the pain, not behind it. Under treatment can occur when surgery patients have a
longer course of recovery than normal: "He's
supposed to be better by now—maybe he's becoming addicted and so pretending not to be
better." For some reason, younger patients are
also generally under treated for pain. You might
call it the "don't-be-a-cry-baby syndrome."

PATIENT VS DOCTOR VS GOVERNMENT

One of the worst impediments to proper
pain relief in a doctor's office is the "paper
chain of red tape" that binds him -- the system
of triplicate prescriptions required for a number
of drugs. One copy of a prescription is retained
by the physician, a second sent to the pharmacist, and the third to the Drug Enforcement
Agency. Triplicate prescriptions are frequently
used to identify physicians who may be "over
prescribing." How a bureaucrat can determine
this, except in extreme cases, by inspecting a
pile of paper is beyond me.

"Over prescribing" of narcotics, stimulants and other drugs <u>accounts for almost 20 percent of the disciplinary actions taken by the Medical Board of California</u> (MBC). The California board and its narc hounds are fanatics on the subject and account for a veritable cornucopia of agony among the citizenry of that state. In 1982, the physician who was then the Medical Board of California's medical consultant declared in an interview sent out to all licensed physicians in California:

"We have two kinds of doctors who get into trouble (for over prescribing narcotics) -- 'script doctors' and 'well-intentioned' doctors. The 'well-intentioned' doctor may appear as a nice guy, but he is really naive or, in some cases, not keeping up with present-day prescribing standards. The 'script doctor' is one who usually knows he is breaking the law and writes prescriptions for controlled substances purely for profit."

It seems to me the higher a doctor goes in medical politics, the more arrogant, ignorant and insufferable he gets.

This interview by the medical board's consultant reflected the traditional view that long-term narcotics use by anyone inevitably leads to addiction. It goes like this: "The body learns to tolerate the drugs and demands ever escalating doses; abuse begins as a search for euphoria, and eventually 'conditioned reflexes' cause an irresistible craving for the narcotic." This pseudo-scientific, Freudian explanation has dominated medical thinking and public health policy <u>for 100 years</u> and is still widely held.

For example, as recently as the June, 1990, issue of the Mayo Clinic's Medical Essay newsletter, they warn: "Opiates can cause drowsiness, nausea, constipation and mood changes. In addition, extended use of opiates can lead to tolerance -- the body becomes accustomed to certain amounts of the drug and no longer responds as well to it. <u>Because of the inevitable addiction that accompanies chronic opiate use, their use in treating pain should be extremely limited</u>." The Mayo clinic should know better and if you go there for surgery, I suspect you may be in for a sticky wicket where pain is concerned. I think you would be better off going to a veterinarian. However, there are some enlightened physicians out there fighting for rational, scientific pain relief -- if you can find one like Kathleen Foley.

"The cancer patient has thus served as a model to demonstrate that opiates can be used on a chronic basis in patients with pain, and this insight has given a greater insight into the clinical pharmacology effects of these drugs," writes neurologist Kathleen Foley in a 1990 monograph on pain management. "For example, chronic use of opiates in the cancer patient has demonstrated that physical dependence occurs, <u>but psychological dependence or 'addiction' is rare, if not nonexistent</u>." (Emphasis added)

A LANDMARK STUDY ON DOCTOR'S ATTITUDES ABOUT PAIN

A 2000 Texas study, with seven researchers from Baylor University and the University of Texas, is probably the most comprehensive study on pain management and mismanagement ever undertaken. It is called: *Physicians' Attitudes Toward Pain and the Use of Opioid Analgesics*. We were so impressed with it that we requested permission from the publisher to reprint it in its entirety. (The tables are in the appendix.)

From your reading thus far in this report, you will not be surprised at the conclusions of the Texas group: "Despite extensive progress in the scientific understanding of pain in humans over the last decade, patients continue to suffer needlessly. Serious mismanagement and under medication occur in the treatment of acute pain and chronic pain. Physicians under treat patients already dependent on opioids and withhold opioids despite evidence that the risk of iatrogenic addiction to prescribed opioid analgesics is low." Actually, this is quoted from the researchers' introduction, but it is also their conclusion.

"Opiophobia" (prejudice against the use of opioid analgesics), was found to be common. And the doctors displayed lack of knowledge about pain and its treatment, and had negative views about patients with chronic pain.

There were some significant findings that I have not seen reported in other studies. Physicians practicing in areas of less than 100,000 population were more fearful of patient addiction and had a more negative psychological profile regarding pain and its treatment than physicians in larger practicing areas.

For reasons not clear (at least to me), psychiatrists had the least negative psychological profile regarding pain and its treatment and tended to be less reluctant to prescribe opioids and less fearful of addiction risk than physicians in other disciplines. The nosayers included the specialties of surgery and anesthesia, where pain is an ever present reality. And keep in mind that the anesthesiologists have set themselves up as pain-management experts!

Frequency Distributions of Survey Results

The various tables in the article reveal some disturbing truths about doctors and pain and we will briefly discuss them here.

Table One -- reluctance to prescribe opioids for chronic pain

Table ONE indicates that health care providers view prescribing opioids as a serious matter, in fact, too serious in most cases. Many feel that a physician is ill-advised to prescribe opioids to relieve the pain of patients with nonmalignant conditions. Overall, 30% of the physicians responding to this survey agreed that opioids

should be restricted to treatment of severe intractable pain, and 10% would withhold opioids
from a patient with severe pain until prognosis
is less than one year or terminal.

This is a disturbing finding and does not bode
well for the patient suffering severe orthopedic
pain, say a debilitated knee or hip, or a sufferer
osf migraine, if he goes to a "Doctor NO," i.e., one
of the unresponsive, uncomprehending and un-
caring 30 percent.

Table Two -- fear of patient addiction

More than 25% of physicians responding to
the survey agreed that any patient who is given
opioids for pain relief is at significant risk of addiction. Nearly 40% would be extremely
concerned about possible addiction if a member
of their family were given morphine for chronic
pain.

Unless the patient has an addictive personality and has demonstrated a tendency for abuse –
with cigarettes, alcohol, tranquilizers and, of
course, narcotics – there is no reason to withhold opioids, including morphine, from the
suffering patient.

Table Three -- fear of DEA scrutiny

The majority of respondents thought there
should be limits to the number of opioid tablets
a patient is prescribed, with almost one fourth
believing that they can avoid being investigated

by giving patients a limited supply of pain medications.

This approach is good politics but bad medicine. Patients vary greatly in their need for pain medication. One- size-fits-all simply doesn't apply here. It is a perfect example of the way government control leads to a Leninist solution to a problem. Half the doctors said they thought the best way to avoid investigation was to avoid using narcotics <u>altogether</u>.

Nearly half agreed that too many opioid prescriptions would lead to external reviews, but that they could avoid investigation "by following the same prescribing practices as other doctors in their field." This is the herd mentality of wildebeests being circled by lions – and you can hardly blame them, but the patients suffer for it.

Table Four -- Knowledge

Most respondents were aware that almost all chronic pain can be relieved with treatment, that the majority of patients having chronic pain are under medicated, and that the best judge of pain intensity is the patient. On the other hand, more than half believed, incorrectly, that psychological and physiologic dependence on opioids (i.e., addiction) is a common result of legitimate prescription. Further, about one third of respondents incorrectly believed that increasing requests for analgesics indicates tolerance to the analgesic, rather than unrelieved pain; disagreed that almost all cancer patients suffer pain;

and disagreed that almost all cancer patients should receive opioids to relieve chronic pain.

Psychological Attributes and the "Medical Model"

The following long quote from this research article describes nicely the psychological dynamics between doctor, patient and undiagnosed pain that demands relief. Dr. Sharon Weinstein said:

"In this study, a disturbingly high percentage of physicians showed negative psychological traits (i.e., authoritarianism, intolerance of ambiguity, reliance on technology, locus of control) regarding patients with chronic pain. Some of these traits can be understood in the context of physicians' practicing under the "medical model."

"In this model, a physician's primary task is determining the cause of a patient's complaint to select appropriate therapy. A complaint leads to diagnosis, which leads to intervention and finally cure. Applying this medical model, a physician is rewarded emotionally for a successful outcome, i.e., "fixing" the problem. <u>Physicians practicing under the medical model are disturbed when they cannot adequately understand the cause of a condition. Without objective demonstration of a pathologic finding, physicians lose confidence and are reluctant to treat</u>.

"Pain management is better understood in the context of a biopsychosocial model. Pain is a complex perceptual phenomenon with both a sensory and an emotional or affective component; as such, it cannot be objectively verified. In managing chronic pain, it is essential to treat patients in a comprehensive manner that encompasses psychological as well as physiologic factors. Some patients require concurrent efforts to manage pain as a symptom while the underlying cause is addressed. In many chronic conditions, pain may become the "disease" or focus of intervention when the pathophysiologic process cannot be identified or effectively removed. "<u>This directly contradicts the medical model, thus challenging the doctor's fundamental principle of practice</u>." (underlining added in all of the above Weinstein quote)

OVERCOMING BARRIERS TO EFFECTIVE PAIN MANAGEMENT

Dr. Weinstein, the lead researcher in the study, summarizes what needs to be done for any real progress to be made:

• <u>Doctors have to make an effort to be aware of personal biases that interfere with clinical judgment</u>.

• Knowledge must be applied in a rational, scientific manner; that is the essence of good clinical practice.

• Current pain treatment guidelines must emphasize thorough pain assessment and

Patients in Pain / 85

multimodal management of this symptom, including aggressive pharmacotherapy.

- A persistent negative attitude toward the patient with pain and bias against opioids as a class of drug must be corrected if these guidelines are to be widely implemented.

- <u>Priority for pain management must be established, equating pain relief with disease treatment</u>.

- <u>Physicians must view pain treatment as important</u>.

- Physicians who choose to participate in [pain programs] may not be those with the most negative attitudes toward pain management, as programs are voluntary.

   <u>Health care facility accreditation organizations are now requiring that pain assessment and relief be monitored as indicators of quality of care</u>." (underlining added)

****

THE MARIJUANA CONTROVERSY

There seems to be a marijuana obsession among some people who should know better. Senator Jesse Helms, one of our finest in my opinion, gave as one of the reasons he opposed the nomination of William Weld as ambassador to Mexico was because he supported the medical use of marijuana. Weld's attitude on the medical use of marijuana was <u>irrelevant</u> and Helm's should have left it out of his explanation for his opposition — Weld was simply unqualified for the job of ambassador. Science and politics makes for a noxious brew of irrationality and bad science.

The Clinton administration allowed so obsessed on the pot issue that they became almost anything (short of a raid on the white House) to prevent even its medical use. The people of the state of California voted overwhelmingly to legalize the controlled medical use of marijuana. The Clinton administration threatened to prosecute any doctor in the state who advises the use of marijuana for pain <u>in spite of the expressed wishes of the voters of California</u>. That's called government by decree, something Genghis Khan was good at.

The National Institutes of Health, the New England Journal of Medicine and The Economist (London) have come out in the support of research on the medical use of marijuana.

Glaucoma, a not always successfully-treated eye disease, has been found to respond with a decreased intra ocular pressure with marijuana use. It is effective in relieving the burning sensations in the arms and legs experienced by some multiple sclerosis patients. And it relieves the nausea from the chemotoxic drugs used in cancer therapy.

Clinton's drug policeman, retired general Barry McCaffrey, scoffed at the idea of using marijuana medically because THC (the active ingredient in pot) has been synthesized and is available as a prescription drug called Marinol. "The argument that this chemical has to be smoked...doesn't make any sense," he said. It may not make any sense to a retired general but what does he know about medicine -- more than the New England Journal of Medicine and the National Institutes of Health? Patients who have tried Marinol say it doesn't work whereas marijuana does. This possibly could be because there is better absorption through the mucous membranes of the lungs or, more likely in my opinion, <u>they haven't synthesized the right chemical</u> from the marijuana.

Marijuana can damage the health, there is no doubt about it. "Cannabinoids" from marijuana smoke is stored in the brain and testes and that's why pot smokers are lousy lovers. And in the case of using pot for glaucoma, it has to be used regularly to maintain the effect. In other words you must stay constantly stoned. After reviewing the medical literature, I am convinced that marijuana has a great future as a medication. Why should anyone be opposed to a rational, scientific investigation of <u>any</u> substance that may help those in pain?

AWAY FROM DICTATORSHIP -- THERE HAS BEEN PROGRESS

Seven states and Washington, DC have approved medical marijuana ballot initiatives, following in the footsteps of California.

In 2000, California voters overwhelmingly endorsed Proposition 36, the "treatment instead of incarceration" ballot initiative that should result in tens of thousands of nonviolent drug-possession offenders being diverted from jail and into programs that may help them get off drugs. "The new law may do more to reverse the unnecessary incarceration of nonviolent citizens than any other law enacted anywhere in the country in decades," says Ethan A. Nadelmann, Executive Director of the *Lindesmith Center-Drug Policy Foundation.*

In Oregon and Utah, ballot initiatives were passed that would have seemed preposterous just 20 years ago -- they require that police and prosecutors meet a reasonable burden of proof before seizing money and other property from people they "suspect" of criminal activity. This is all well and good but what about the hundreds -- maybe thousands -- of people across the country who have been stripped of everything they possess -- often including their children? They are penniless and so unable to prosecute for the return of their possessions. Their money has disappeared into the coffers of local and federal government and the pockets of the crooks who run these programs.

"No doubt many of them were guilty," is the frequent reply. No doubt, but is it the American way to catch five, or even ten dealers, and destroy even one innocent family?

These two states went a step further and mandate that the proceeds of legal forfeitures be handed over not to the police and prosecuting agencies who had seized the property but rather to funds for public education or drug treatment.

Even more encouraging is the actual decriminalization of marijuana use in over a dozen states. People are coming to their senses as they see their neighbor carted off to jail in handcuffs. One county in California, Mendocino, approved a local initiative to decriminalize personal cultivation of modest amounts of marijuana. And in 1998, Oregon re-jected an effort by the state Legislature to re-criminalize marijuana.

People are digging in their heels, realizing that the drug "war" has become an excuse for coercion, terror, intimidation and outright rob-bery. I don't know if these measures will work, but they are a start. The corruption is so intense and pervasive, at all levels of government from the county to the White House, that it may be too late. As Mr. Nadelmann said:

"The struggle over implementation of the initiative in California has already begun, with many of its opponents trying either to grab their share of the pie or to tie the process up in knots. Powerful vested interests in the criminal justice business, accustomed to getting their way, did not look kindly on the challenges the proposi-tion posed to the status quo."

Ref: Los Angeles Times, 2000
       Ethan A. Nadelmann, Executive Director of the
       Lindesmith   Center-Drug   Policy   Foundation,
       <*www.drugpolicy.org*>

THE UN SUPPRESSES ITS OWN REPORT ON POT

Aging hippies, with their now gray pony tails and pot belies, lugged signs in the 60s pronouncing that pot was safer than alcohol or tobacco. This was a self-evident falsehood to most Americans (including me) and we enjoyed seeing them bashed and imprisoned. They were a threat to our culture and our liberties. While this "threat to our culture" is true in a broader sense, the hippies were right on the comparative safety of marijuana. New Scientist, is a respected science magazine that appeals to a wide audience of scientists and people in the university graduate class of every stripe, from psychology to biology. According to a document leaked to New Scientist, the analysis concludes not only that the amount of dope smoked worldwide does less harm to public health than alcohol and cigarettes, but that the same is likely to hold true even if people consumed dope on the same scale as these legal substances (which they don't).

The comparison was due to appear in a report on "the harmful effects of cannabis" in December 2000 by the World Health Organization. The report was suppressed following a long and intense dispute between WHO officials, the cannabis experts who drafted the report, and a group of "disinterested" advisers.

As the WHO's first report on cannabis for 15 years, the document had been eagerly awaited by doctors and specialists in drug abuse. The official explanation for excluding the comparison of pot with legal substances is that "the reliability and public health significance of such comparisons are doubtful." However, insiders say the comparison was scientifically sound and that the WHO caved in to political pressure. It is understood that advisers from the US National Institute on Drug Abuse (NIDA) and the UN International Drug Control Program (IDCP) warned the WHO that "the report would play into the hands of groups campaigning to legalize marijuana."

Of course the report would have "played into the hands" of those wanting to legalize marijuana. But suppressing the report, i.e., suppressing the latest scientific findings on pot, also "plays into the hands" of those who have a tremendous interest in the continuing drug war, no matter how futile it has been proven to be – bureaucratic dictatorships just love organizations like the IDCP and the NIDA. They help the bureaucrats maintain control over us sheep with a cover of pseudo science and double talk.

One member of the expert panel which drafted the report, says: "In the eyes of some, any such comparison is tantamount to an argument for marijuana legalization," which, of course, it is. Another member, Billy Martin of the Medical College of Virginia in Richmond, says that some WHO officials "went nuts" when they saw the draft report.

Remember "scientific-bureaucrat" is an oxymoron. They are not interested in the truth. It reminds one of the Pearl Harbor tragedy. The American people were not told that Roosevelt had planned in great detail, for at least two years, the specific bombing of Pearl Harbor with the entire fleet, except the carriers, bottled up and defenseless. Thousands of deaths were a foregone conclusion.

What is the point of this Pearl Harbor betrayal story? The point is that Roosevelt started the war by strangling the Japanese economy and forcing them to attack us in desperation. The American people, who were overwhelmingly against the war, were too stupid to realize that World War II would be good for them. It would be good for the economy and would save the world from the bad guys. At the world wide cost of 100,000,000 dead, the economy was indeed saved but the bad guys – Soviet Russia and Soviet China --won anyway.

It has become clear that the present "war on drugs" is destroying the nation and this type of deception and censoring of science will produce results worse than Pearl Harbor.

The section that was extirpated from the report was open and reasonable. As reported by New scientist, the leaked version of the excluded section states that the reason for making the comparisons was "not to promote one drug over another but rather to minimize the double standards that have operated in appraising the health effects of cannabis." "Nevertheless, in most of the comparisons it makes between cannabis and alcohol, the illegal drug comes out better -- or at least on a par--with the legal one," reported New Scientist.

The report concludes, for example, that "in developed societies, cannabis [pot] appears to play little role in injuries caused by violence, as does alcohol." It also says that while the evidence for fetal alcohol syndrome is "good", the evidence that cannabis can harm fetal development is "far from conclusive."

The report says that while heavy consumption of either drug can lead to dependence, only alcohol produces a "well defined withdrawal syndrome," i.e., clinical evidence of addiction. Heavy alcohol consumption can lead to cirrhosis, severe brain injury and a much increased risk of accidents and suicide. None of this is true of pot and there is only "suggestive evidence that chronic cannabis use may produce subtle defects in cognitive functioning."

Cannabis fared better in five out of seven comparisons with alcohol in long-term damage to health. (Underlining has been added to the New Scientist report.)

You may be wondering, what with my fervent defense of pot legalization, if your reporter is himself a pot head. I tried it twice and I inhaled both times. I tried a few puffs about 1980. It made me feel paranoid and fearful -- not a pleasant experience at all. The next time was at a wedding party in 1992. I had no mental reaction at all but I developed a cough which took three weeks to clear. I don't like pot but if someone wants to smoke it, it's none of my business, none of your business, and none of the government's business. Your government, with its ruthless destruction of our liberties and property rights in pursuit of marijuana dealers and smokers, is far more dangerous than pot. With Pearl Harbor, the Japanese turned their guns on us. With the "drug war," we are turning our guns on ourselves.

Ref: New Scientist, 21 February, 1998

ADDICTS VS PATIENTS IN PAIN

Many addicts claim to have been hooked on drugs during medical care and older studies indicated perhaps 10 percent of addicts started off that way. However, a major study in 1980 showed abuse developed in only 4 of 11,882 patients given opiates while hospitalized; in only one instance was the abuse considered major.

In recent years, self-infusion pumps have been introduced which allow patients after surgery to give themselves limited doses of narcotics to control pain, as mentioned above. It has been a God-send <u>when it is used</u>, which isn't often enough. There were fears that the process would create "a new population of drug addicts." Instead, <u>the amount of narcotics used by patients has been the same or less than under the old PRN method</u>. This is because a patient in pain with even half a brain quickly learns when he needs the narcotic and will administer it, thus preventing getting "behind the curve" and thus requiring a bigger dose than is necessary when the pain is caught in time. It can be compared with infection and antibiotics: the earlier in the infection the antibiotic is started, the less it will take to cure it.

There is a major difference between addicts seeking <u>euphoria</u> and individuals seeking <u>relief from pain</u>. The traditional perception is that the reactions of street addicts are simply a more extreme expression of what happens to chronic pain patients. But there is a major difference. Drug addicts behave as though obtaining and using drugs are primary drives, like eating, sleeping or sex. They take drugs to get high and are frequently lost to themselves, their families and society -- the drug is all that matters. When a patient is in extreme pain, the drug is also all that matters, but the objective is different. The person with chronic pain takes drugs to return to normal and to get on with a normal life. The addict has no conception of what a normal life is, or he has forgotten.

Unlike an addict, <u>the typical pain patient experiences little or no euphoria from narcotics</u>. It seems that euphoria is "traded" for pain relief. (This isn't always true however.)

Withdrawing from drugs is a major hurdle for addicts, but for the pain patient withdrawal is quick and typically uncomplicated.

There is now a redefinition of the key terms of drug abuse. All long-term users of narcotics become physically dependent: if drugs are suddenly discontinued, their bodies react with sweating, aches, nausea or other withdrawal symptoms. That physical dependence was <u>once thought virtually synonymous</u> with addiction, but is no longer. The American Society of Addiction Medicine now defines addiction as the abuse of any psychoactive substance <u>with compulsion and loss of control despite adverse consequences</u>.

Similarly, an American Medical Association Task Force describes addiction as a chronic disorder characterized by "the compulsive use of a substance resulting in physical, psychological or social harm to the user <u>and continued use despite the harm</u>." "Psychological dependence," which emphasizes the compulsive use of drugs, is now often used interchangeably with the term addiction. This in no way defines the typical hospital patient in pain. After the body has healed, drugs are forgotten, no matter how much narcotic they had during their ordeal. So when a patient would come to my office claiming that he was addicted due to a severe illness or injury and so it was the doctor's fault, he was an addict, in my view, until proven otherwise. With this AMA Task Force report, I see a ray of hope.

Under the older definition, anyone who became physically dependent could be viewed as an "addict" -- including the pain patient on narcotics. The newer definition distinguishes between the pain patient trying to escape pain while healing and the self-destructive addict trying to achieve euphoria or "getting laid" as one of my street-wise addiction patients once described it.

DOCTORS UNDER ATTACK

Even a supposedly safe practice -- giving narcotics to terminal cancer patients — is under attack. This humane approach, a part of a doctor's "raison d'être", is sometimes criticized for placing medical care "nearer to euthanasia." In a well-publicized case in 1990, the morphine-related deaths of two terminally ill patients in the Minneapolis area were ruled by the coroner to be homicides. I wonder how many cancer patients will have to live out their final days in agony in Minneapolis because of this ruling. (Don't take this to mean I am recommending euthanasia. We have enough trouble playing Marcus Welby without playing God.)

There is constant pressure for more discipline of physicians. A recent example is a draft report of the US Department of Health and Human Services which says data strongly suggest "the universe of potentially actionable events far exceeds the number of disciplinary actions actually imposed by the (state) boards." In other words the Washington bureaucrats don't think enough doctors in the US (or in the universe) are being prosecuted for over use of narcotic drugs.

As usual, the patients are the losers in this meddling. Physicians are aware of the ongoing disciplinary actions against doctors for "over prescribing" drugs, usually narcotics. As a consequence, many physicians simply limit the amount of narcotics they will prescribe for any one patient in pain. Some physicians even shy away from using any triplicate forms at all. The forms are a paperwork nuisance and a red flag of danger. Not having them is also a convenient excuse for not treating pain patients. This is a form of abandonment, brought on by government meddling in the practice of medicine.

Doctors shy away from patients who complain of chronic pain. Pain patients often appear normal, so it's difficult to determine the extent or validity of the complaints. The patients are often querulous, manipulative (you would be too if you had to lie, cheat, steal, and prevaricate to get pain relief) and depressed. High levels of medication to relieve pain, which these patients often need and demand, invite disciplinary problems for the treating doctor.

Most physicians prescribe narcotics only for chronic pain patients they have treated for a number of years. Patients receiving such medication face a major problem if they move to a new area or their physician retires. New physicians will be extremely reluctant to treat them. Essentially, they have been "orphaned." The following case is a perfect and tragic example.

This is the case of a 26-year-old athlete who sustained a major spinal injury that caused him to suffer from excruciating pain in the back and legs. The pain rendered him unable to work, and he became a burden to himself, his family and society, which pays his medical bills. His physician discovered that small doses of morphine taken orally each day (the way cancer patients receive them) obliterated the pain. With the help of the medication, the young man resumed working and made plans to marry his childhood sweetheart, who was accepting of his injury.

One day, however, the physician was accused by his regional medical association of prescribing narcotics for a purpose unapproved by the association and of turning the patient into an addict. Fearful of losing his medical license, the physician stopped prescribing the drug. (Where morphine administration is allowed by law, physicians can technically prescribe it at will, but they are in fact restricted by the regulations of medical societies and state pharmacologic boards which control licensing.)

Of course, the young man's pain returned. In desperation, he turned to other physicians and was rebuffed. He then sank rapidly into depression and again became mired in helplessness and hopelessness.

The Texas Legislature confronted the under prescribing problem in 1989 by enacting a law which defined "intractable pain," added to state law language from federal law, recognizing the legitimate medical use of "dangerous drugs," and the existing over disciplining of physicians treating chronic intractable pain -- another ray of hope.

It has always irritated me that doctors are quick to give "<u>mental</u> narcotics,"-- tranquilizers, anxiolytics, mood elevators, words with no scientific meaning -- to women (mostly) for their mental "problem." A gynecologist, for example, will "treat" his patients with these drugs *although he knows little or nothing about the physiology, addictionology or toxicology of these dangerous chemicals.* And he is encouraged to prescribe these drugs by a nice young man – and now, increasingly, attractive women --in a business suit who has been sent in by the pharmaceutical company to teach the doctor the wonders of their particular feel-good drug. The addictions from these agents can be <u>very painful</u> when the withdrawal commences. Paxil, for instance, one of the en vogue tranquilizers, can take you <u>to the pits of hell</u> when you try to take your life back by abandoning this fearful master. The drug salesmen know little or nothing of this. And the doctor who has caused this terrible problem, <u>usually never hears about it</u> because the patient goes to <u>another</u> doctor to get off the addiction. (She probably figures that if the doctor was ignorant enough to get her addicted to such a drug, then he probably isn't smart enough to get her unaddicted -- and she is probably right.)

Neurotic patients are prone to have additive personalities and so they are the last people who should be prescribed tranquilizers. The prescribing doctors, usually unqualified in the use of these life-destroying chemicals, can induce an incapacitating addiction in a patient and he will not be punished. In fact, no one will complain about it, not even the patient. The unwritten law seems to be that it's the patient's fault if she becomes addicted. The doctor was only trying to help; she was an "addictive personality" and so now she must pay the price. It never seems to occur to them that if the patient was an addictive personality, the drug was <u>contraindicated</u> in the first place..

Yet, these same doctors can face revocation of their medical license and even imprisonment if they were to induce an addiction in an attempt to relieve a patient's suffering from physical pain, even the pain of terminal cancer. Because of the drug war (a completely failed war with consequences far more horrific than the failed war in Viet Nam) doctors now have their hands tied in the treatment of pain. It is a great national tragedy that control of pain has been turned over to bureaucrats and narcotics agents such as your friends in BATF and the FBI, the people who brought you the Ruby Ridge murders and the Waco killings. Would you rather trust your doctor's judgment in relieving you of your suffering or the people at the Bureau of Alcohol, Tobacco and Fire Arms?

One of the greatest errors in medicine today is the belief that patients in severe pain will become addicted to narcotics as you increase the dosage to relieve the pain. Another part of that error is the belief that the dose of narcotic will have to be continually increased as the patient becomes inured to its effects and that this "tolerance" will eventually make the narcotic ineffective, even at very large doses. The third part of this trinity of error is that large doses of narcotic will cause respiratory depression and death.

None of these perceptions are valid <u>if the patient is in severe pain</u>. The body, by means not understood, "burns up" the narcotic as it is used, <u>if it is being used</u> <u>for its intended purpose</u>, the relief of pain, and not for recreation. There will be <u>no</u> respiratory depression, <u>no</u> addiction and <u>no</u> level of ineffectiveness because of repeated usage. The research is unequivocal on the relationship of pain therapy and addiction — <u>there is none</u>.

Morphine is God's gift to the terminal cancer patient. Morphine and Demerol were, until recently, the <u>only</u> medications that would stop the terrible suffering. (Fentanyl, a relatively new narcotic, will be discussed later.) But the paranoid governments, state and federal, have not only cracked down on drug dealers and users (ineffectively), but on the doctors (very effectively.) So to relieve your suffering, you must convince your doctor to risk imprisonment by going to the streets for your drugs, or you must move to Mexico -- or kill yourself.

PAIN PATIENTS ARE NOT -- AND WILL NOT -- BECOME ADDICTS

A study in the *New England Journal of Medicine* found that of <u>11,882</u> hospital patients with severe pain who were treated with narcotics, only <u>four</u> became addicted. That's .03 percent — about one in 3,000. A 1982 survey of 10,000 burn patients who were treated with narcotics for pain found an addiction rate of <u>zero</u>. Yet, bone-headed bureaucratic zealots are combing doctor's offices, especially pain specialists, looking for violations. Frank Adams, a pain specialist in Texas has remarked: "Drug agents have been turned loose <u>and are totally out of control</u>. They do not know how to discriminate between the legitimate and illegitimate use of these drugs. <u>This is police-state medicine</u>." (Emphasis added)

The president of the Future of Freedom Foundation, Mr. Jacob G. Hornberger, remarked on the developing police state in America: "(Americans) cannot bring themselves to face the terrible truth: that their own government has become an organization of state terrorism...it is still too nightmarish for the average American to accept. His mind simply will not assimilate and process the data." Nowhere is this more evident than in the oppression of doctors and their patients and the cruelty resulting from this tyranny.

Unfortunately, doctors have never seen pain as a priority in the treatment of patients. Patients will often suffer untold agony following surgery because the control of pain is an afterthought to the surgeon if he thinks about it at all. I can attest to this from a personal experience. (It would be helpful if every doctor could go through a severe pain experience before being issued a license to practice.) I had an exploratory operation on my right wrist following an injury. The surgeon, a gentle and caring man, promised me that he would order an IV drip of Demerol following the surgery because the pain would be severe --since it would be added to the excruciating pain I already had. I felt good about this because, like everyone else, I do not enjoy pain.

I awoke from surgery with the feeling there was a trip hammer in my wrist pulsating at the rate of my heart. There was no Demerol drip; he had forgotten. So, you see, being a doctor does not guarantee you from suffering. Once you are horizontal in a hospital bed, you're just another member of the suffering masses. And remember, this was the behavior pattern of a basically caring and gentle person. I don't understand it. Maybe they think you <u>have</u> to be in pain so they'll know you're still alive. Maybe it's the respiratory depression myth but, whatever it is, this attitude among doctors was extant even <u>before</u> the current hysteria and paranoia about drug addiction, in fact, way before.

Even the Catholic church, not known for making hasty decisions, has stated, through Catholic scholars, that "suffering has no special purpose in the divine scheme." Isn't that <u>great</u>? You no longer have to suffer your way into heaven. You can just walk right through the gate. BUT, there is a little problem; the doctors haven't caught up with the thinking of the Catholic church and pain remains unimportant to them, something you have to endure. So unimportant, in fact, that there is <u>no mention of pain</u> in the Encyclopedia of Medical History, 1985!

Going back just a few generations in this sorrowful tale of patients and their pain, we come to the man who did more to separate physicians from reality than anyone else in the history of medicine, Sigmund Freud, who should be renamed Sigmund Fraud. Sigmund so transformed medical thinking that patients were changed from people with real problems to suspected neurotics. This was reinforced a few generations later with the advent of laboratory testing which could confirm or deny whether the patient had a "real" problem or was one of the many "Freudian" neurotics who only thought he was sick and in pain. But, as any honest doctor will admit, you can be extremely ill, and in pain, and still have perfectly normal blood laboratory values. One of the many disciples of the degenerate cocaine enthusiast, Sigmund Freud, one Georg Groddeck, said that all pain was, at bottom, psychological. If you had a kidney stone, a broken leg or a gunshot wound to the chest, how would you like to have him for a doctor?

In the mid 19th Century, Harriet Martineau complained of dreadful abdominal pain but her doctors could not make a diagnosis and so left her in misery for the rest of her life with no further attempts at diagnoses. Today, with surgery no longer tantamount to a death sentence, the doctors eventually would have done an exploratory laparotomy -- opened the abdomen to take a look. They may have found mesenteric adenitis, a benign swelling of the lymph nodes of the abdominal cavity, or they may have found nothing. In any case, the modern medical mind is little different than what it was 150 years ago. The conclusion would be: "We couldn't find anything significant so the pain is not justified and so there is no treatment justified." If there is no name for the condition, then no condition exists. Sir Thomas Beddoes remarked: "A language has not yet been adjusted with any degree or exactness, to our inward feelings." In other words, <u>The Name of the Game is the Name</u>." If you can't call the signs or symptoms of the patient by a name, it doesn't exist. Harriet's pain didn't exist -- except "in her head."

The real tragedy here is that a simple solution was at hand even back in 1850, at least from Harriet's point of view. The doctors cared about the diagnosis; Harriet cared about the pain. They should have given her a powerful narcotic to see if it relieved her pain, simple as that. If it relieved the pain, and Harriet was not an addict, then the pain was real. Is that so difficult for a professor of medicine to understand? They should have given her an injected placebo of normal saline first. If that relieves the pain, then you have a good case for "mental illness," whatever that term may mean.

Even philosophers have attacked the reality of pain as though it didn't exist except in the patient's mind. The distinguished French surgeon, René Leriche, said that "pain serves little purpose either diagnostically or prognostically; indeed in certain chronic cases, it seems to be the entire disorder which, without it, would not exist." I wonder how many patients, living in misery from chronic pain, would like to give René a not-so-gentle twist of a thumb to see if they could persuade him to look a little deeper into the subject of pain.

The Leriches of the world are still with us. Jeffery Bernard, a columnist for the London spectator, has experienced not one but two of life's most terrible versions of the devil's dish — acute pancreatitis and "phantom limb." Phantom limb is a condition where the patient experiences severe pain in a limb that has been amputated, for instance, pain in the foot but the foot is no longer there. Bernard had some choice words for British doctors: "...most of all I hate them for their meanness and narrow-mindedness about dispensing pain relief."

A final word on the patients-will-become-addicts controversy by a distinguished judge.

This little item is on the "indomitable human spirit" -- the right to destroy your own life without government help. These unfortunate self destructors comprise only <u>slightly more than one percent </u>of the population. The other 98.7 percent -- including you and me -- are not, and never will be addicts, even if the drug war was abandoned tomorrow and we could buy heroin at the local news stand.

Despite billions spent to wage war on drugs... and a prison population that is the envy of incarcerators the world over... federal judge John L. Kane noted that "about 1.3% of the population is addicted to cocaine - the same percentage as in 1979, a few years before the Drug War, <u>and the same percentage as in 1914</u>, when cocaine was sold legally in grocery stores."

Ref: the Independent Institute

PART II

PEOPLE IN PRISON

"...it is difficult to escape the conclusion that, notwithstanding the contrary evidence of impressive scientific and technological achievements, we stand once again knee-deep in a popular delusion and crowd madness: the Great American Drug craze." -- Thomas Szasz, MD [From *Our Right to Drugs* -- Greenwood Publishing Group, Inc., Westport, CT]

PROHIBITION – IT STILL DOESN'T WORK

Most doctors don't withhold narcotics from patients just to be mean although, as Bernard found out, it can appear that way. It's more a matter of indifference, fear (of government regulators) and ignorance of the way narcotics work in patients experiencing severe pain. To be fair, but not to excuse them for their desertion of patients in pain, doctors are, like their patients, victims of the insane "war on drugs." <u>Americans didn't learn a thing</u> from our first experience with prohibition. That moral crusade, led by the amoral force of government and adelpated, self-righteous women, had a predictable result: a dramatic <u>increase</u> in drinking, immorality, corruption in government, gambling and prostitution. It gave us a greatly expanded Mafia and arrogant billionaire bootleg families such as the Bronfmans in Canada and the Kennedys in America.

Critics can say that's hindsight and this is true. If I had been an adult in the twenties, I might have approved of prohibition (though I doubt it). But the average American today doesn't even seem to be able to use hindsight. He doesn't see that today's corruption and degeneration -- up to and including the White House and the Congress -- are caused only partially by the <u>use</u> of drugs but more by the <u>prohibition</u> of drugs. If we should have learned anything from the early 20th Century, it was that <u>prohibition doesn't work</u>. People have the constitutional right to kill themselves with alcohol or drugs or anything else. Government moral crusades always lead to corruption -- and the end of freedom. Lenin and Hitler both led "moral" crusades against capitalism and "other exploiters of the people."

This book was not meant to be a diatribe against the prohibition of narcotics. But the more I got into the problem of pain, the more I realized that <u>the pain problem for patients cannot be solved until this unconstitutioal prohibition, like the previous one against alcohol, is stopped</u>. This is a touchy subject because many people who understand the enormity of the current <u>power abuse</u> in the name of curbing <u>drug abuse</u> are afraid, if they speak out, of being labeled as left-liberals and thus bracketed with the abortionists, the tree-huggers and the animal-loving asp-kissers who think nothing of letting their dog give them a nice lick on the lips just after they have licked their genito-urinary system. (Who would want to be identified with <u>those</u> people?)

In fact many of your fellow Christians will turn their backs on you in the misguided belief that you are, somehow, "supporting" drug abuse. But is it Christian to support a war that is directed against Christianity as well as all the other decent aspects of our country? Can Christianity survive in a dictatorship? Ask the people of China and Cambodia.

I confess that, for many years, I was for the "drug war." Drugs were going to destroy our youth and thus destroy our country. But drugs are not going to destroy the country; <u>the government</u> is going to destroy the country in the name of preventing drugs from destroying the country. Drugs <u>may</u> destroy the country but if I have a choice between a drug-free, Stalinist police state and putting up with some junkies on the streets, I will take the junkies. Most addicts, if left alone, don't bother anybody. The DEA, the BATF and the FBI are bothering <u>everybody</u>, and making millions of innocent people live -- and die -- in pain because of the spillover of the "drug war" into the doctor's office and the hospital.

This "spillover" concept was the central thesis of this book until I realized that the two problems were inextricably bound together. The government drug warriors are fighting drug dealers, drug users and innocent patients. Psychologically and legally, it will be impossible to solve the patient abuse problem without the complete legalization of narcotics.

Have there been any positive results from "the war on drugs?" From the Washington Times, front page headline: "Experts See signs of Drug Epidemic" -- Not just an increase but a drug epidemic. The National Center on Addiction and Substance Abuse did a survey and found the following: Seventy-six percent of high school students and 46 percent of middle school students said drugs were present at their schools. More than a quarter of high school students said that a student died in their school from drug overdose within the last year. Thirty-five percent of students surveyed said drugs were the most important problem they face -- up from 31 percent in 1996.

THE KISS OF DEATH -- GOVERNMENT EDUCATION ON DRUGS

While extreme, a recent BBC show in England illustrates a growing resentment against government intrusion in matters of what we eat, what we drink or, even, what we inject. It was a special report on drugs in Britain. The report be-littled the danger of addiction from drugs, which is what the kids want to hear. But there was a lot of truth in the report, from the stand-point of exaggeration of the addiction problem.

Taking cannabis, cocaine, ecstasy and even heroin is not dangerous but extremely enjoy-able, according to the program. Smoking a cannabis joint is as relaxing as drinking a glass of wine, while many people find taking ecstasy the most pleasurable experience of their lives. Injecting a modest dose of heroin can make mundane but essential household chores enjoy-able, drug users said.

The headline, *HEROIN IS SAFE AND FUN*, is preposterous and irresponsible journalism be-ing presented to a gullible audience not needing any more excuses to act irresponsibly. The mes-sage was, as I interpreted it, "A lot of teenagers and adults are using drugs but most of them end up leading normal lives." <u>This is true</u>, but we are reluctant to admit it. And the message would come through: "OK experiment with drugs while you are young; you'll grow out of it."

However, because television is the molder of the mass mind, and nothing short of abolish-ing TV will solve <u>that</u> problem, we have to keep pressing the issue of dangerous addiction and ruination of life, <u>even though it may not be as bad as claimed in the press and the educational</u>

institutions. Will this hypocritical approach
work? Obviously it hasn't as the DARE program
has proved. The kids saw through it and drug
use has rocketed.

The presenter, Mat Southwell, is a former
NHS employee who says he has taken ecstasy for
12 years, and still does so regularly. He enjoys
drugs and argues they should be legalized. "Most
people take drugs because they want to relax and
feel good, much in the same way they might have
a drink at the weekend. But while alcohol is so-
cially acceptable, people are being put in prison
for the chemical equivalent of buying a round of
drinks," Southwell said.

One user on the program explains: "Heroin
is my drug of choice over alcohol or cocaine. I
take it at weekends in small doses, and do the
gardening." Fair enough, it's his life, but is this
the message we want delivered to impression-
able children?

"The program was lambasted as irresponsible by John Griffith, chief executive of the
group *Drug Abuse Resistance Education* (DARE),
which works in 500 schools to warn children of
the dangers of drugs," the Observer reported.
DARE is everywhere! And everywhere, proves
its futility. The number of illegal drug-takers in
Britain has risen from around a million in the
Sixties to three million in the Eighties, and to
around 10 million now. Would it be extreme to
say that DARE has made the problem worse?

Why can't people see that government coercion, or even just government persuasion, <u>is the primary problem</u>, not the answer. DARE will be discussed in more detail, as it relates to the U.S., in the next chapter.

In the UK, all drugs were legal, and used routinely across society, until 1860. <u>The former Prime Minister William Gladstone and Florence Nightingale used opium, while Queen Victoria used cannabis</u>. These three worthies would agree with the director of the show.

Mat Southwell said it's a simple matter of human rights: "'The principle of individual freedom linked to social responsibility lies at the heart of our democracy. As an adult and responsible member of society I absolutely assert my right to take any mind-altering substance, be that ecstasy, alcohol, heroin, tobacco or cannabis. No one, least of all the state, has the right to tell me otherwise."

In 1860, the temperance ladies took over and everything was banned but alcohol and tobacco. The result has been disaster: When cocaine was criminalized, global production was about 10 tons a year, but it has since swelled to 700 tons a year. <u>Illegal drugs now account for eight per cent of global trade, making it one of the three largest businesses in the world -- along with oil and the arms trade.</u>

THANK YOU, LADIES!

Ref: Sunday Observer (London) 3/25/01, Anthony
    Browne

****

What's going on here? We expend billions of dollars to fight the "war" and we have a disaster on our hands. If I'm wrong for opposing the drug war, please explain to me why.

Explain to me why the Chicago Tribune is wrong. In the following excellent article from the Tribune, there is some annotation by this author [in brackets.] All underlining was added.

Prohibition: Self-Righteous Self-Destruction

"Here's a maxim for the times: Policies of Prohibition create drive-by shootings. Whether the perpetrators were tommy-gun wielding minions of gangsters like Al Capone, or are the Uzi-toting gangbangers of today, drive-bys mostly are driven by the brutal requisites of the underground economy.

"In other words, much of the violence plaguing too many inner-city communities is directly connected to the Prohibitionist policies that pump profits into drug dealing. The anti-alcohol forces of old had overwhelming public support; they even managed to push through a constitutional amendment to the Constitution to aid their crusade. But the public soon realized Prohibition was bad public policy. The social damage caused by attempts to prohibit booze far exceeded the damage done by drinking alcohol. Our present war on drugs is bad public policy for the same reason.

"However, drug prohibition has had far more destructive consequence than our foolish adventure in constitutional teetotalism. In addition to empowering elements of organized and unorganized crime, fueling violence and the corruption of public officials, the drug war also has justified the diversion of resources to criminal justice agencies at the expense of other needs.

"For instance, U.S. drug policies have created an incarceration rate that leads the world, accelerated the environmental ravages caused by crop eradication programs and triggered military intervention in countries more in need of economic aid. What's more, the drug war's unconscionable assault on civil liberties threatens to trash the Constitution's most hallowed protections.

"But unlike during the Roaring '20s, the domestic price of these misguided policies is disproportionately being paid for by the African-American community. Last month Human Rights Watch published a report that found black drug users are imprisoned at many times the rate of white users in this country (57 times the rate of whites in Illinois).

"It was the latest study in a growing library of data revealing wide racial disparities in the drug war's casualty rate. The racially skewed enforcement of drug prohibition identifies African-Americans (and to a lesser extent, Hispanics) as the primary targets of drug warriors. Perhaps that's why so few politicians publicly question the manifest failures of our drug policy.

[This does not mean that racial profiling is not necessary under the present system, since most of the street dealers are of the Negro race. But the cold, hard truth is, these blacks are expendable in this phony war. There are always more to replace those you have put in prison. When you capture the new group of dealers, the original group will be released as there are not enough prison cells to hold them all. When the first group is recaptured, well, you get the picture -- a revolving door policy has been established that is good for the prison industry. In the meantime, the top echelon of drug dealers are rarely apprehended -- and they are primarily hispanic or white. -- Ed]

"A report issued by The Justice Policy Institute found more failure: one in four prisoners are behind bars because of a non-violent drug offense. Since 1980, the study notes, the number of violent offenders entering state prisons has doubled, the number of people imprisoned for drug offenses has increased 11-fold. According to the study, entitled "Poor Prescription: The Costs of Imprisoning Drug Offenders in the United States," we will pay more than $9 billion to keep 458,131 drug offenders behind bars this year.

"Among the study's most notable facts are that a majority of drug offenders are imprisoned for <u>simple possession</u> of drugs; the U.S. imprisons 100,000 more people for drug offenses than the entire European Union jails people for <u>all</u> offenses, even though the EU has 100 million more citizens than the U.S.; those states with the highest incarceration rate of drug offenders also have the highest rate of drug use; between 1986 and 1996 the number of whites imprisoned for drugs doubled, for young blacks it increase six-fold.

[In the first two lines of the very long sentence above, there is an important issue that has escaped most people. <u>If it took a constitutional ammendment to force liquor prohibition on the American people, how have they managed to force drug prohibition without using the same constitutional process</u>? Keep in mind that the 18th Amendment, as so cogently described by Dr. Thomas Szasz, did not prohibit the <u>drinking</u> of alcohol, or even the <u>possession</u> of alcohol. Even the promoters of the Volstead Act did not attempt to control American's personal habits as it, clearly, would be an act of tyranny. The 18th amendment only restricted the <u>transportation</u> of liquor.

"...deep in their hearts," said Dr. Szasz, "they...realized that a competent adult in the Land of the Free has an inalienable right to ingest whatever he wants. It should be unnecessary to add...that there was no question, during prohibition, of randomly testing people to determine if there was any ethanol in their system, or of

searching their homes for alcohol, or of imprisoning them for possessing alcohol, or of
involuntarily treating them for the 'disease' of
unsanctioned alcohol use."]

"'The war on drugs has never been a war on
drugs per se." noted Barry Holman of The Justice Policy Institute, "It has always been a war
on people...'

"But the social costs of the suicidal drug
war are becoming more apparent and a growing number of Americans are beginning to balk
at paying it. An initiative on the ballot in California would substantially reduce the
incarceration rate of drug offenders and fund
an additional $120 million in drug treatment.
A drug-reform initiative, proposed in New
York by the state's chief judge, would provide
treatment rather than imprisonment for 10,000
addicted offenders.

[Forced treatment is a Soviet concept and
will only create another bureaucracy living off the
weaknesses of the human race. Government cannot legislate successfully against bad personal
habits. We learned nothing from the disastrous
Volstead act. -- Ed.]

"These are minor alterations to be sure, but
they represent important breakthroughs in the
battlefield mentality that is relentlessly pro-
moted by drug war propaganda."

"The biggest change may be taking place in
the African-American community, whose lead-

ership finally is beginning to question the value of drug prohibition. The issue of drug decriminalization increasingly is listed as an item for discussion at civil-rights conventions and other activist gatherings.

"Although most of our politicians refuse to admit it, Prohibition's time has passed--again."

Ref: *Chicago Tribune*, 7/31/00, Salim Muwakkil [Reprinted with the kind permission of Mr. Muwakkil.]

***

I can't spend anymore time on this. My readers will get cranky and say I'm getting carried away again with my anti-government paranoia, which is true (Douglass Aphorism # 6: "If you don't think the government is after you, then you haven't waited long enough, or you are part of the problem.")

Let me recommend a short but extremely cogent article on this subject by the assistant editorial page editor of the Las Vegas Review-Journal, Vin Suprynowicz. It appeared in the November, 1996, issue of Freedom Daily. A copy of the issue containing this article will set you back two bucks and may change your thinking on the drug "war." If it changes your thinking, then being the intelligent, forceful and influential person that all of my readers are, you may change the world. See the references at the end of this book for ordering instructions.

Go to the video store and rent the movie, *Traffic*, staring Michel Douglas. This is a very gritty, brutal movie and not for the faint of heart. Most women will probably walk out of it because most women can't face reality. (I am not faulting them for this; this is a man's job -- and BOY, have they mucked it up.) The message in the movie is clear: THE WAR ON DRUGS IS LOST AS CLEARLY AS THE WAR IN VIET NAM WAS LOST.

After you have read what the judge has to say in Appendix IV and the other excellent pieces in the Appendix, and you have seen the movie, tell me what YOU suggest.

I have taken on this battle against the "drug war," -- a ploy for the total enslavement of the American people -- with great hesitation. It took me <u>ten years</u> to make up my mind and I have with considerable trepidation -- I don't want my Christian relatives and friends to think I have deserted the principles of my ancestors. But I have come to the conclusion that it is <u>not Christian</u> to support a drug war that is a far greater threat to our liberties and our faith than the original alcohol Prohibition, Communism or Nazism.

In (partial) defense of the doctors, the New Prohibition has made "Trading-With-the-Enemy suspects" of any doctor using narcotics for his patients. By that I mean, if the doctor is giving "too much" narcotic, he is helping the illegal drug traffickers and is some how profiting from this "traffic", i.e., "trading with the enemy" – <u>even though the drugs he is prescribing for the patient are perfectly legal</u>! I'll tell you a personal story so that you can see the extent of the paranoia and frenzy of control that has gripped us in the field of narcotics in the treatment of patients.

In the early nineties, before I fled to Russia to escape the medical tyranny that was obviously descending upon "the land of the free," I was treating cancer patients in the mountains of north Georgia. Many of these patients were in pain and so required narcotics in order to make life bearable. A certain druggist in the village in which I was practicing didn't like my politics, my method of practice or anything else about me, including my <u>dog's</u> politics. Feeling a strong sense of civic pride and a desire to protect the imbecillic public from charlatans such as me (and my dog, Liberty), he contacted the Georgia Board of Pharmacy and told them I was "prescribing large amounts of narcotics to out-of-state patients," the implication being there was some kind of interstate dealing in drugs involving patients, pseudo patients or other undesirables.

I had a visitation from a nice lady from the state board of pharmacy. She was a law school graduate, probably a young grandmother, quite pleasant and almost apologetic. She said that she was aware of my work, was a subscriber to my newsletter and, after investigating the allegations, had found nothing wrong with my prescribing patterns. I thanked her and assumed that was the end of the matter.

A patient took a prescription for Percodan, a strong form of codeine that is addicting to those using it as a recreational drug, to a pharmacist in Savannah, Georgia, and he refused to fill it because, he said, "there was some question" about my prescribing habits. That was 200 miles from my office! How could he know about the "prescribing habits" of an obscure doctor 200 miles away? My conclusion was that I had been betrayed by the nice lady from the state bureaucracy and I was on a "hot list," of drug-dealing suspects without the slightest evidence that this was true — all based on the action of one pharmacist who didn't like to see a doctor deviating from the state-sanctioned (and enforced) guide lines for pain control. How many doctors are going to risk their license to practice medicine to help patients in pain under these circumstances? I closed the office and moved to Russia where there is still a modicum of freedom in medical practice.

Although your doctor is carefully-controlled and watched for the slightest deviation in his use of pain medications, illegal drugs are everywhere. Two separate studies have found that over 80 percent of the money in circulation tests positive for cocaine. Yet, as a doctor I can no longer purchase medicinal cocaine for the treatment of migraine headaches. This treatment, called a spheno-palatine ganglion block, is the most effective treatment for migraine headaches ever devised. It not only stops the current headache but prevents their return, often for months or years. But medicinal cocaine has simply disappeared and so millions must suffer, thanks to the "war on drugs."

To understand why you and your doctor can't work together to relieve your pain, you've <u>got</u> to understand the terrible police state that has developed in this country in the name of fighting drugs. Unless drugs are legalized and the government, at all levels, is forced to give up its insane and paranoiac war on the American people, you may soon be facing a situation where, to relieve your pain, you will have to take to the streets and buy narcotics from a dealer who may very well be a narcotics agent working on the side. (Then you will endure your pain in jail – and <u>really</u> be neglected.) Your alternative (after you get out of jail) will be to just suffer -- or move to Ecuador and chew beetle nuts. (Which, I am told, isn't a bad idea, under the present political circumstances. Beetle nuts are an excellent pain reliever.)

The virtuous Mr. Bill Bennett, our former drug "czar," has recommended suspending constitutional rights to fight the drug "war" and <u>public beheadings </u>of drug dealers. *Bennett The Virtuous* viscously attacks those who oppose his

Muslim approach to the drug problem. He calls them "intellectually and morally scandalous."

Let's look at the people Bennett sees as "intellectually and morally scandalous": Bill Buckley, James Bovard, Thomas Szasz (one of the few psychiatrists in the world who conservatives would trust), Representative Doctor Ron Paul (THE number one defender of American liberty in the House of Representatives, he is called "Doctor No" by left-liberals who hate his unwillingness to compromise his principles.) and Nobel Laureate Milton Friedman. Who is this haughty hypocrite, Bennett, to challenge the morality and intellectuality of these men? Look in the mirror, Bill. Write a letter of apology to these sincere and patriotic Americans and plead for their forgiveness for your scurrilous remarks.

And while you are at it, ask the American people for their forgiveness for your reckless, immoral, and intellectually-bankrupt "war" that has become a war on American liberty as the drug problem has <u>escalated</u>.

In 1989, Los Angeles police chief Daryl Gates recommended that drug <u>users</u> "be taken out and shot." The National Guard is now actively at war with the American people. There is a National Guard Bureau in Washington and under that bureau is something called the Drug Demand Reduction Section (DDRS). I don't understand exactly what that weird title means but

I know what it means to the chief of that section of our new police state — "attitude change" of the American people at the point of a gun.

The National Guard, under the zealous direction of one Colonel Richard R. Browning of the aforementioned DDRS, entered in 1992, without a warrant, more than 1200 private buildings and trespassed on private property more than 6500 times. According to The Pittsburgh Press, "80 percent of the people who lost property to the federal government were never charged with a crime." Most never get their property back and some people have been killed during attempted property seizures. The dedicated Colonel Browning, feels that the National Guard is the ideal agency to make some "attitude changes" in the American people. He says that "...military force must be used to change the attitudes and activities of Americans who are dealing and using drugs. The National Guard is America's feasible attitude-change agent." Attitude change at gunpoint? Beheadings? Shooting drug users? Do you smell the vapors of tyranny here or do you have a sinus problem?

It was only 80 years ago that we drank of the bitter drought of alcohol prohibition. This forced morality was not unconstitutional, as some people think, because the Congress and the people can make anything constitutional by amending the document, such as the power to

make the drinking of alcohol a government-certi-
fied sin or, if they like, outlawing the eating of
meat, the smoking of cigarettes, the eating of al-
mond seeds and prohibiting making naughty
remarks about some group that you don't like
such as the Hairy Krishna, the Princess Di Memorial Fan Club or the Zionists. But it's OK to make
naughty remarks about home schoolers, Palestin-
ians, Arabs in general and white males. Now
things have gotten so out of control that Clinton
and his gang changee the law at the stroke of a
pen and <u>even ignored the diktats of the Supreme Court</u>. The Extreme Court, now a
nine-man dictatorship, thought it had control of
this country until the Clinton crowd came into
power. Can't you just hear Bill Clinton asking,
when the Court objected to one of his unconstitutional acts, "How many troops does the Supreme
Court have?"

I have digressed, so now back to Prohibition. Finally, once it was realized that alcohol
prohibition was counter productive and leading
us to a state of anarchy more or less controlled
by rum-runners, politicians and the police
themselves, the amendment was repealed. <u>But
now we are repeating this terrible crime against
ourselves</u> because they who experienced the
tragedy of prohibition are dead and few Americans read history. If you go back and read the
pious polemics of the alcohol "reformers," all
you have to do, to bring the sermon up to date,

is substitute for the word "alcohol" with the new buzz word and enemy of the people: "DRUGS."

WHAT IS TO DONE?

We are headed straight down the road to total bureaucratic dictatorship very similar to the nazi state of Adolph Hitler. The signs are there; everything is in place:

Random searches of people and their property

Confiscation of property without due process -- police regularly and use filched goods to pad police department accounts -- and their own pockets

Character and racial profiling methods

Going around the laws, the Congress and supreme court rulings

Military-like attacks on homes and businesses with commando gear and semi-automatic weapons

Constant anti-drug propaganda exceeding anything Joseph Goebbels could have contrived

Paid informants -- everywhere in every type of business, including your bank, the post office, the hospital and soon -- if Bush gets his way in getting the government into your church with cash -- your own church will not be a safe haven from the prying eyes of the drug thugs and the IRS.

Forced treatment by psychiatrists, psychologists and other brain parasites, no different than the methods used by Stalin against political dissidents.

Rampant bribery -- Unlimited funds are available to bribe the bribeable. As was pointed out in the superb movie on the drug war, *Traffic*, the drug lords have far more money to fight their side of the drug war than does the federal government. This sounds preposterous but keep in mind that the various agencies of the executive branch can only spend what the Congress gives them. It is not possible to appropriate that much money. They can out spend us ten or twenty to one.

Terror tactics -- if you are a bank teller and suspect drug money is involved in a transaction (with not a shred of evidence), and you do not report it, YOU are liable for prosecution for misprision of a crime if they nab the suspected miscreant -- you're are in the clink with him. In fact YOU WILL BE EASIER TO CONVICT THAN THE SUSPECT. He fits a profile for drug dealers taught to you; there was a large cash transaction; he was too charming and loquacious. You should have recognized these "signs" and turned him in -- and you didn't. If you had turned him in, you would be a free and respected citizen, not a felon facing a jail term.

And further more, you would have received a nice cash reward -- a bounty -- for doing your

<u>duty</u>. Who would not give in to this? If you don't <u>over report</u>, you're jeopardizing your self, your family, your job -- your whole future. If you go to jail, you become a felon, you can't vote; you can't obtain a weapon-carry permit, you can't leave the country <u>and you would not be allowed to work in a bank</u> or any other type of job -- a guard for instance -- where you must be bondable -- for YOU are no longer bondable.

Are you smelling the vapors of tyranny yet? If not, you must have a sinus infection.

PART III

PATIENTS IN PAIN
-- HOPEFUL SIGNS

The paradox of modern scientific medicine's inhumane approach to pain, i.e., ignore it, was highlighted in a report from the Memorial Sloan-Kettering Cancer Clinic. Drs. Foley and Sjernswaard reported from the Second International Conference on Cancer Pain:

"Under medication continues to be the major problem in the United states, despite excellent studies showing that the psychological dependence characteristic of addicts almost never develops in pain patients. Patients with cancer pain easily discontinue their drugs when the source of their pain is removed...

"Nevertheless, drug use and drug abuse are so inextricably linked in the public mind that even physicians continue to believe opiates have the power to transform...patients into addicts. Over the past 15 years, researchers... have gathered an impressive body of data showing that effective pain control, far from causing addiction or heavy sedation, permits many patients to function better."

The New Prohibition, which makes enemies of the doctors and "prisoners of pain" of the populace, has many unrecognized casualties including most surgical patients who are denied pain relief. Scientific American stated in 1990: "Society's failure to distinguish between the emotionally-impaired addict and the psychologically-healthy pain sufferer has affected every segment of the population. Perhaps the most distressing example is unnecessary pain in children."

According to Dr. Richard Blonsky, president of the American Academy of Pain Medicine, Up to 70 percent of terminal cancer patients do not get enough pain-relief medicine. Dr. Russell Portnoy, director of analgesic studies at Sloan-Kettering Hospital, New York, said in 1987: "The under treatment of pain in hospitals is absolutely medieval."

A major study released in 1996 involving 9,000 patients at five medical centers showed that about half the patients died in pain. In thousands of cases, doctors disregarded living wills and other advanced directives.

Because of the government's paranoia about drug addiction, and their intimidation of doctors whom they now control more than any other profession or group, patients in pain are being abandoned by doctors. This is unprofessional conduct of the worst sort. The doctors should revolt against the state and federal bureaucracies and refuse to follow edicts that keep their patients in pain. There wouldn't be a Dr. Kevorkian making headlines about helping patients to commit suicide if the doctors were performing their duty to their patients who are in pain. Is Kevorkian the only doctor left with any courage? I do not agree with Kevorkian but he at least was willing to go to jail in order to stand up for what he believes.

Even experts in pain management, like Dr. Kathleen Foley, have to simply watch cancer patients suffer because the amount of oral medication they need for pain relief for a month exceeds the state's legal limit. Part of the irony of this, says Dr. Foley, is that the oral opiates, such as Demerol and morphine, "don't have much value as street drugs."

Patients themselves have contributed to the phobia concerning narcotics. All patients, like most doctors, think that morphine is invariably addictive. Even parents of children suffering from cancer are often more concerned with the addictive potential of the drug than with its pain-relieving effects! And telling elderly outpatient cancer patients that they are being given a "strong" drug for their pain, often results in their not taking the drug at all. Imagine being so fearful of addiction that you will endure awesome pain to avoid an addiction that you don't have and won't get.

There is such a fear of morphine addiction that one pain specialist has proposed that morphine be renamed in order to overcome the resistance to this extremely effective blocker of severe pain. This won't work, of course, unless the <u>doctors</u> start thinking realistically about the use of narcotics in relieving suffering. A Hungarian physician who practiced in Hungary for 60 years, was way ahead of his time. He told his cancer patients that he was giving them "sal thebaicum," and he never used the name morphine. His patients probably lived longer, I would guess — and they died in peace.

Dr. Sandon Saffler, medical director of a California hospital, represents the mind set of the average doctor on the matter of pain. He repeats the usual myths about addiction and increased tolerance to narcotics and concludes: "The best approach may be to send the sufferer to a pain clinic where various treatments can be tried to see what works best."

Anyone familiar with these clinics knows what that means — the use of practically anything except that which works best -- narcotics -- because "everyone knows that pain-killers are dangerous and create addiction, tolerance and respiratory depression." This does not mean that acupuncture, hypnosis, "counseling" (usually by someone who has never experienced real pain), electrical methods, magnets and the like should not be tried. But I can guarantee you these non-drug methods <u>are not going to work for patients with terminal cancer</u>. These patients do not need magnets; they need meperidine. They do not need counseling; they need codeine. They don't need massage; they need morphine. Anything less is simply inhuman yet, it is the norm.

When "the war against the war" reaches the cover of TIME magazine, you know that progress is being made (*The Case for Morphine*, APRIL 28, 1997). Logo"Although TIME doesn't go the last mile and call for the cessation of the drug war, they at least call for the rational use of narcotics for the suffering patients of America.

"No one is advocating the use of narcotics to treat a stubbed toe," TIME says. "These powerful drugs are indicated only for the most severe, disabling pain. But research conducted over the past 20 years into the mechanisms by which the body experiences grievous pain suggests that certain narcotic drugs are so well suited to relieving suffering that it seems callous, maybe even negligent, not to use them."

This is strong stuff from middle-of-the-road TIME. I hope the doctors are listening. (This article was written years ago and it seems to have had no lasting effect on the doctors. Here is the reason why:

TIME remarked on the marked difference in medical use of narcotics by the various states:

"That doesn't mean a doctor can prescribe narcotics with impunity. For one thing, this can be hazardous to one's career. Medical-review boards in some states, notably Tennessee, West Virginia and New York, are notorious for singling out physicians who prescribe a lot of narcotics and yanking their licenses. "I tend to under prescribe instead of using stronger drugs that could really help my patients," a West Virginia doctor admits. "I can't afford to lose my ability to support my family."

Don't get seriously sick or injured in Tennessee., West Virginia or New York.

FINALLY, LEGISLATIVE HELP

California State Senator Green has taken notice of this atrocious gap in medical practice: "Quite frankly, I am outraged by the unwillingness of the medical profession to wake up and join the 20th Century." He has written a law that lifts the threat of punishment from doctors who prescribe painkillers for people with intractable pain. Green is so outraged by the inhumanity of it all that he wants to go even further and <u>fine or jail doctors</u> who do not live up to their Hippocratic oath and relieve suffering with appropriate narcotics.

I thought Senator Green was going too far until I read the pathetic story in Otto Scott's Compass newsletter about Alma Herrington. Alma fell and injured her spine. She sustained a compression fracture and a ruptured disc. <u>She had a total of six back and spine operations</u> and got no pain relief from any of these surgeries -- that's more pain than the suffering of Jesus on the cross. She is now disabled and in constant pain and <u>the doctors have refused to prescribe narcotics for her</u>. Alma Herrington is, of course, encouraged by Green's attempt to help her and other sufferers through legislation: "It's not just me," she said, "There are thousands of people like me out there. We are dehumanized, stripped of all pride and dignity." Otto Scott expresses well these same sentiments in his article on pain in the January, 1997, issue of Compass:

"The idea that cancer patients should receive pain killers only in the terminal stage of their slow deaths is simply barbaric. To have to argue for such relief on their behalf is almost unbelievable. The idea that sufferers of illness should be left to suffer, when inexpensive and thoroughly known relief is available, is inconsistent with our technological age."

OK, Senator Green, you win; I'll support your bill. The only problem is that, with your legislation, the state narcs will put some doctors in jail for "over prescribing" (in spite of your law) and they'll put others in jail for "under prescribing" (because of your law.) Pretty soon most of the doctors will be in jail, in court, or out on probation, terrorized that they may prescribe too much or too little. Your law <u>doesn't go far enough.</u> We must get rid of this New Prohibition by getting the states and the federal government <u>out of the drug business entirely</u>.

MAKING PROGRESS AGAINST THIS SUI-CIDAL WAR

We have by no means won the defensive war we are fighting against our <u>own government</u>, the "War on Drugs," but the tide is turning toward sanity and reality. <u>We will never win back all of the liberties we have lost</u> from this terrible war against the American people. It doesn't work that way. Just as in all the wars we have fought since the American revolution, "emergency measures" are imposed without the consent of the people. After the emergency has passed, at least half of the unconstitutional laws are retained. This present internal war of Washington <u>and the states</u> versus the American people will be the <u>most debilitating of all of our wars</u> with the possible exception of the insane war of the North against the South, 1861-1865.

"Election day 2000 was a big day for drug policy reform.

In California, voters overwhelmingly endorsed Proposition 36, the "treatment instead of incarceration" ballot initiative that should result in tens of thousands of nonviolent drug possession offenders being diverted from jail and prison into programs that may help them get their lives together. The new law may do more to reverse the unnecessary incarceration of nonviolent citizens than any other law enacted anywhere in the country in decades. But don't

count on it. The governments agents are powerful and ruthless and they will not relinquish
power easily.

"It wasn't just California that opted for drug
reform. Voters in Nevada and Colorado approved medical marijuana ballot initiatives,
following in the footsteps of California, Oregon,
Alaska, Washington state, Maine and Washington, D.C. In Oregon and Utah, voters
overwhelmingly approved ballot initiatives requiring police and prosecutors to meet a
reasonable burden of proof before seizing
money and other property from people they
suspect of criminal activity--and also mandating
that the proceeds of legal forfeitures be handed
over not to the police and prosecuting agencies
who seized the property but rather to funds for
public education or drug treatment.

"These were not the only victories for drug
policy reform at the ballot in recent years.
California's Proposition 36 was modeled in part
on Arizona's Proposition 200. In Oregon, the
first of 11 states to decriminalize marijuana during the 1970s, voters in 1998 rejected an effort
by the state Legislature to recriminalize marijuana. And in Mendocino County, Calif., voters
this year approved a local initiative to
decriminalize personal cultivation of modest
amounts of marijuana.

"Clearly, more and more citizens realize that
the drug war has failed and are looking for new

approaches. The votes also suggest that there are limits to what people will accept in the name of the war on drugs. Parents don't want their teenagers to use marijuana, but they also want sick people who could benefit from marijuana to have it. People don't want drug dealers profiting from their illicit activities, but neither do they want police empowered to take what they want from anyone they merely suspect of criminal activity. Americans don't approve of people using heroin or cocaine, but neither do they want them locked up without first offering them opportunities to get their lives together outside prison walls.

"So what do drug policy reformers do next? In the case of medical marijuana, three things: enact medical marijuana laws in other states through the legislative process; work to ensure that medical marijuana laws are effectively implemented; and try to induce the federal government to stop undermining good-faith efforts by state officials to establish regulated distribution systems."

The above five paragraphs are from Mr. Nadelmann's report to the Los Angeles Times in November, 2000. Mr. Nadelmann is falling into an old trap here. As Dr. Thomas Szasz has so clearly pointed out, <u>drugs need no regulation at all</u>. As with alcohol, drug use is none of the government's business, state or federal. In San Francisco, you can purchase a bottle of liquor in any convenience store or grocery store and their problems in California are no better or worse than those in any other state. In the following paragraph, Nadelmann seems to grasp what the actual outcome will be with the politicians and bureaucrats still left at the levers of power in this otherwise productive legislation.

"...The struggle over implementation of the initiative in California has already begun, with many of its opponents trying either to grab their share of the pie or to tie the process up in knots. Powerful vested interests in the criminal justice business, accustomed to getting their way, did not look kindly on the challenges the proposition posed to the status quo.

"If California's new law is implemented in good faith, with minimal corruption of its intentions, the benefits could be extraordinary, saving taxpayers up to $1.5 billion in prison costs over the next five years while making good drug treatment available to hundreds of thousands."

Mr. Nadelmann, sincere as he is, does not seem to grasp the fundamentals of "political science." Few laws are passed with "good intentions;" they are passed to increase the power of the lawmakers and their friends down the food chain of power. There will not be "minimal corruption" of the intentions of the bill but maximal corruption. Freedom is the only system that works and there will be no freedom in the drug situation so long as the

government has any part in it. Leaving "education" and "treatment" in the hands of the same
government power brokers is doomed to fail.

"Proposition 36 also provides a model--both
for initiatives in other states where public opinion favors reform but the legislature and/or the
governor are unable or unwilling to comply,
and in states like New York, where no ballot initiative process exists to repeal draconian and
archaic laws. The initiative victories demonstrated once again that the public is ahead of
the politicians when it comes to embracing
pragmatic drug policy reforms. Yet there was
also growing evidence this year that even some
politicians are beginning to get it. Three states--
North Dakota, Minnesota and Hawaii--legalized
the cultivation of hemp (to the extent permitted
by federal law). Hawaii enacted a medical marijuana law this year, with the support of Gov.
Ben Cayetano."

Mr. Nadelmann's conclusion is encouraging,
almost inspiring -- and I wish him luck in this
critical battle for freedom:

"Perhaps it's too early to claim that all this
adds up to a national vote of no confidence in
the war on drugs. But the pendulum does seem
to be reversing direction. Call it a new anti-war
movement. Call it a nascent movement for political and social justice. Or simply call it a
rising chorus of dissent from the war on drugs.
The election results have made it clear that drug

policy reform is gaining momentum--in California and across the country."

Ref: Los Angeles Times, 11/26/00

> Ethan A. Nadelmann is Executive Director of the Lindesmith Center-Drug Policy Foundation (www.drugpolicy.org), a drug policy reform organization.

THE DEATH OF DARE

The pathetic history of DARE is a classic example of why Ethan Nadelmann's approach to the drug war is only half right i.e., pushing the bureaucrats out at one end of the system and then building their power base at the other. Ironically, this bureaucratic and wasteful chimera was created in California, a state sincerely trying to solve it's problem without grasping the critical fact that government IS the problem, not the solution.

DARE is the acronym for Drug Abuse Resistance Education. The education program is a complete multi-million-dollar failure and is being consigned to the Dempster Dumpster by an increasing number of schools.

The propaganda blitz was so effective that DARE metasticised to every state in the union and Great Britain, as related above.

Los Angeles Police Department chief Daryl Gates, a loose cannon on the deck of law enforcement if there ever was one, conceived of DARE. A better explanation for the acronym would be: Drugs Are the Reward of Empire, as the empire, the drug enforcement behemoth of the government, has been richly rewarded with the complete powers of the police state and DARE has done its share.

Gates, undoubtedly dedicated to the "war on drugs," but under armed in logic, education and common sense, hit the ramparts with all guns blazing. Before any reasonable defense could be devised, he had captured most of the schools in America. In 20 years, he has gained the control of over 20 million young minds, wasting their time and energy and dramatically increasing their interest (and usage) of drugs. These policemen-turned-social-workers (no doubt sincere but out of their element) are toiling in every state and in three-quarters of the nation's school districts. Armed with Mary Calderone's sex education (how-to-do-it courses) and the inane Gates drug education (Just Say What?) young Americans are prepared to march bravely forward in this brave new world -- and into the pit of self-indulgence.

America is deluged with DARE paraphernalia — including bears, bumper stickers, buttons, hats, and jeeps. DARE has everything — except good results. Only in America can so much money be spent for so little -- DARE is the mirror image of the public school system itself.

The federal Bureau of Justice Assistance paid $300,000 to the Research Triangle Institute (RTI), a North Carolina research firm, to analyze DARE's effectiveness. The RTI study found that <u>DARE failed significantly to reduce drug use</u>. Researchers warned that "DARE could be taking the place of other, more beneficial drug-use curricula."

For $300,000 I think they could have been a little more forceful; something like: "DARE is a dud -- <u>toss it</u> and put the police back on the street."

"Suburban students who participated in DARE reported significantly higher rates of drug use... than suburban students who did not participate in the program," reported Dennis Rosenbaum, professor of criminal justice studies at the University of Illinois at Chicago.

From a California study: the Los Angeles Times reported: "...DARE didn't keep children from using drugs. In fact, <u>it found that suburban kids who took DARE were more likely than others to drink, smoke and take drugs</u>."

Salt Lake City Mayor Rocky Anderson recently denounced DARE as "<u>a fraud on the people of America</u>." Mr. Anderson, who yanked DARE from Salt Lake City schools, complained: "For far too long, drug-prevention policies have been driven by mindless adherence to <u>a wasteful, ineffective, feel-good program</u>. DARE has been a huge public-relations success but a failure at accomplishing the goal of long-term drug-abuse prevention."

The power brokers at DARE, puffed up with their power and sense of immunity to criticism, sued Rolling Stone for libel for having the temerity to tell the truth about their pathetic feel-good program. It blew up in their faces, like an exploding cigar, when the judge ruled that there was "substantial truth" to the charges that DARE had sought to "suppress scientific research" critical of DARE and "attempted to silence researchers at the Research Triangle Institute, editors at the American Journal of Public Health, and producers at 'Dateline: NBC.' " This was a stunning defeat for this inanely silly and destructive program.

As author James Bovard summarizes it: "DARE's feel-good photo opportunities are no substitute for effective drug education. American children deserve something more than a drug program that fails to persuasively inform and warn them of the danger of narcotics. Politicians, school officials and police need the courage to admit DARE is a dud."

James Bovard is the author of *"Feeling Your Pain: The Explosion & Abuse of Government Power in the Clinton-Gore Years"* (St. Martin's Press).

PART IV

SOME PROMISING TREATMENTS FOR PAIN

MAGNETS – PAIN RELIEF OR QUACKERY?

Carlos Valbona, M.D., a rehabilitation medicine specialist at the Baylor College of Medicine (Texas), had scoffed at the idea of magnets applied to the skin relieving pain. But more and more patients were coming in and telling him the magnets worked on their particular pain.

His curiosity was finally aroused to the point that he started dabbling with the treatment, even though he was aware that the words "magnet" and "quack" had become synonymous among those who deride alternative medicine in the press.

His first patient was a priest who had post-polio back pain so severe he couldn't lift his hand to bless his parishioners. "I told him, 'There is one thing I could try. It hasn't been proved scientifically, but it might just help,' "

Dr. Valbona said to reporter Judith Mandelbaum-Schmid, *a contributing writer at Walking* magazine. He placed one magnet on the priest's back. "Within minutes," says Valbona, "he came out of the examining room and said: 'It's a miracle. I can raise my arm.' "

Encouraged by these results, Valbona undertook a study of fifty subjects, half of whom would receive a placebo for their pain (a dummy magnet) and the other the magnet therapy.

76% of the magnet-treated patients reported pain relief during the 45-minute treatment period, compared to only 19% of the placebo patients. These findings in a double blind study are really impressive. Do they really work? Patients think so. Americans spent an estimated $200 million on magnets in 1998 alone and other universities have followed Valbona's lead, reports Judith Mandelbaum-Schmid, Running Magazine. Among them:

Ronald Lawrence, M.D., an assistant professor of psychiatry at the University of California, Los Angeles

Paul Rosch, M.D., President of the American Institute of Stress

Robert R. Holcomb, M.D., Ph.D., an assistant professor of pediatrics and neurology at Vanderbilt University School of Medicine

Michael Weintraub, M.D., neurologist at New York Medical College

Brad Worthington, M.D., Vanderbilt University

John Parziale, M.D., a clinical assistant professor of medicine at Brown University in Providence

With an array of talent like that, I don't think magnets will be equilibrated with quackery much longer.

If magnets relieve pain, and they certainly seem to, no one knows how they work. Some experts believe magnetic energy alters the chemical interactions in nerve fibers that are responsible for pain impulses. Others say the effect is due to increased blood flow to the area (I subscribe to the first theory.)

Action to take if you want to try magnetotherapy:

A magnet is a magnet so one is as good as the other as long as you have the proper strength. The magnet should be 500 to 1,000 gauss. The best place for you to start is with *the North American Academy of Magnetic Therapy*, 800-457-1853

They will send an information package to you with product recommendations, and a referral service to physicians who perform magnet therapy.

Ref: Judith Mandelbaum-Schmid, Running Magazine

* * * *

There is another ray of hope for pain relief. I don't know why hope always comes in rays but this particular ray, if used for the suffering, could be a step forward in rational pain relief. A raspberry-flavored lollipop (and a lozenge form) loaded with a narcotic pain-killer for treatment of cancer patients has been recommended for federal approval. The recommending body is a Food and Drug advisory panel that voted <u>unanimously</u> for clearing the drug.

The question came up that a child might get custody of a narcotic lollipop and we know where <u>that</u> would end — a dead child and a law suit. The drug in the lollipop, fentanyl, can be fatal to children. But this obvious circumstance can happen with any drug, including baby aspirin. As a nurse member of the panel said: "Some kid, somewhere, somehow, is going to do this (eat the lollipop). But do we deny this benefit to cancer patients for that reason?" This drug, Fentanyl, is a relatively new narcotic and has proved to be very well accepted by terminal cancer patients in severe pain and, in fact, advanced Cancer Patients Prefer Fentanyl by patch to oral morphine.

A cohort of patients with advanced cancer were studied at University of Sheffield where they found that the use of transdermal fentanyl was preferable to sustained-release oral morphine, though both treatments appeared to be equally effective. "Transdermal" means to apply to the skin as with a patch. The application of the lollipop to the mucous membrane of the mouth will work the same way only faster. The reason for the Fentanyl preference was that constipation and daytime drowsiness occurred significantly less frequently with use of the fentanyl patch than with use of oral morphine. There was, however more insomnia with the Fentanyl patch.

A REMARKABLE ANESTHETIC DISCOVERY

If confirmed by repeat studies, a sensational advance in surgical safety has been discovered. It has been reported in the *British Medical Journal* (BMJ), from research in Australia, New Zealand and the UK, that an epidural anesthetic before major surgery can cut the risk of dying <u>by as much as a third</u>.

An epidural anesthetic is an injection of one of the "caine" drugs, such as Lidocaine, into the "epidural space," which is the compartment on the outside of the sheath that covers the spinal canal. It is a safe procedure in competent hands and is used often in deliveries.

According to the report, epidurals also reduce the chances of patients suffering a range of complications from pneumonia to blood clotting in the deep veins, which may lead to fatal emboli (clots) to the lungs—the dreaded

pulmonary embolism. The study of 9,500 patients produced amazing statistics:
- respiratory depression – cut by 59 percent
- pulmonary embolism – cut by 55 percent
- clotting in the veins – cut by 44 percent
- pneumonia – cut by 39 percent

Since pain is one of the great neglected areas in medicine (See my book, A Painful Dilemma – the Dilemma of Pain), this discovery has enormous implications. Although it has been known for years that a pain-free patient heals quicker with fewer complications, little has been done about it. Pain management has often been an afterthought with surgeons and anesthesiologists alike.

The researchers give credit to "altered coagulation, increased blood flow, improved ability to breathe free of pain, and reduction in surgical stress responses" for the good results obtained. While all of these may be significant, I would give maximum credit to pain relief, no matter where the pain is located. Pain is debilitating; it kills your appetite; it lowers your ability to heal. It is no exaggeration to say: "Pain kills."

Action to take:

If you are facing surgery, ask your surgeon if he plans to give you an epidural along with the usual anesthesia. If you draw a blank, send him a copy of this article. Unless he is a complete bonehead, he will see the reference at the bottom of this article and take the appropriate action.

Ref: British Medical Journal, 12/15/00.
Clifford Woolf, M.D., Ph.D., anesthesiologist, Harvard Medical School

The so-called "super aspirin," the COX inhibitors, have created a lot of optimism in the pain field. Gastritis and other side effects have, from the first aspirin, limited the use of oral pain killers. You take the pain-killer and then you must take another pill to neutralize the side effects of the pain medicine. While many people can take almost any form of medicine with impunity, a large percentage cannot. We are in the age of one-size-fits-all medicine -- "Take two capsules twice daily, or as directed by your doctor."

This approach is farcical. If John weighs in at 350, and Mary at 100, will they get the same dosage of medication? Often they do, but dosage is only a small part of the problem. Recent research has revealed there are <u>hundreds</u> of ways that people differ from one another. For efficient and effective -- and safe -- medication, each drug must be tailored to the physiology of the patient. <u>And this is coming soon,</u> to a drug store near you.

I know it sounds like science fiction but drug companies do not put billions of dollars into science fiction, at least not on purpose. We are very critical of drug companies because of their sloppy research, obfuscation when caught in a mistake, their greed rather than attitude of service to mankind and their promotional methods -- especially the direct promotion of drugs to the public. There have been notable 20th Century advances, without a doubt. The antibiotics, insulin, diuretics and, well, those are the only ones I can really get excited about.

Ironically, the drug companies may, because of genetic advances, turn out to be a boon to mankind after all. But for the time being, we are stuck with OSFA drugs (One-Size-Fits-All) and so we will report to you some modest advances in the OSFA field.

There is a new class of NSAIDs that can curb pain without plaguing users with gastrointestinal problems. Known as COX-2 inhibitors, these new prescription drugs work in essentially the same way as older NSAIDs, such as aspirin and ibuprofen, by blocking prostaglandins. But COX-2 drugs are targeted to affect only prostaglandins that cause inflammation and pain while leaving alone those that protect the lining of the stomach and small intestine, regulate kidney function, and help govern blood clotting. If they work out as billed, they will be a boon to pain sufferers.

Magnetic resonance imaging (MRI) and positron emission tomography (PET) have enabled doctors to look in on the brain and measure, to some extent, how continuous pain can lead to damaging changes in both the brain and the peripheral nervous system that then make suffering even worse.

Neuropathic pain is a real horror because there is no fully effective pain reliever for it and it is the worse pain known to man. NSAIDs have no effect on such pain. Opiates and "adjuvant analgesics," drugs that were not designed for pain relief, including anticonvulsants, antidepressants, and sodium channel blockers, have pain-relieving properties but can only blunt neuropathic pain, not relieve it.

"At the moment," says Clifford Woolf, M.D., Ph.D., an anesthesiologist at Harvard Medical School, "there is no good specific treatment for chronic pain, and clinics are filled with people desperate for relief....But now that we're beginning to understand how we perceive pain, we can identify what people are suffering from and design appropriate therapies. I'm optimistic that we'll see significant advances in the near future." I think Dr. Woolf is correct but not for anything reported here. Genetic engineering is the key to complete pain relief, just as it will be for the cure of many diseases.

Some other innovations are controlled-release pills, which slowly dispense medication into the bloodstream over the course of 8 to 12 hours rather than the more customary 3 hours. Transdermal patches, like those used to help wean smokers off nicotine, can deliver drugs through the skin, <u>bypassing the gut altogether</u> if stomach problems are a problem. Certain opioids can now be provided in metered doses with an inhaler, making medication easier to take for patients who have difficulty swallowing and, again bypassing the digestive tract. And small pumps can be surgically implanted in the body to deliver drugs directly to the circulatory system or spinal canal, with the dose controlled by the patient or from a nursing station.

Ref: *New Choices: Living Better After Fifty*, March, 1999, Richard Laliberte

PART V

FINDING PAIN RELIEF WITHOUT A DOCTOR

If you have severe pain that is different from anything you have had before, you should see a doctor. You are not qualified, although you may be a brilliant physicist, astrologist or palm reader, to determine the seriousness of your pain. For instance, a pain at the right upper quadrant of your abdomen may be gall bladder inflammation, appendicitis, kidney stone, colitis, pneumonia or even early shingles. These things require the services of a qualified doctor because all of them (except shingles) can be "fixed" with proper medical or surgical care. When in doubt about pain, see the doctor.

There are a number of simple and effective things a person can do for acute pain problems but most people are unaware of them and doctors in general don't think about them. Acute soft tissue and musculo-skeletal injuries for instance: ankle and wrist sprains, back aches from lifting, contusions (bruises,) should be treated immediately after the injury with cold compresses, using ice if possible. This is to quiet the tissues down and limit the degree of swelling. Twenty minutes, every two hours for the first 12 hours is about the maximum benefit to be expected from this phase of the treatment.

After the first 24 hours, heat, wet or dry (I prefer wet but I can't tell you why; it just seems more effective to me than a heating pad) is applied to encourage the migration of healing cells, prostaglandins and enzymes to the injury site. An ancient doctor-philosopher once said: "I trust a hot towel more than I do most doctors."

With an infection, such as a boil on your nose, go immediately to heat -- ice will be of no avail. I have found that most superficial infections of the skin can be cleared up quickly with this simple method and save you a lot of misery, including surgical incision of boils — not a pleasant experience. For a boil, I recommend very hot compresses every two or three hours at first. When you begin to see (or feel) an improvement, cut back to three times a day. Each treatment should be for thirty minutes. If you are sensitive to the heat and feel that you are "cooking" your skin, then you probably are. Cut back on the intensity of the heat and/or the length of the treatment. In other words, use common sense.

For pain, always consider color therapy. It can be surprisingly effective. See my monograph on color therapy (*Color Me Healthy*) which is available from RHINO PUBLISHING, S.A. at 1-888-317-6767 or Int'l + 416-352-5126. Visit my website at www.drdouglass.com for more information.

Acupuncture, TENS (electrical stimulation through the skin), chiropractic, massage and hypnosis all have their place in chronic, musculo-skeletal pain management.

If all of the above fail, plus phrenology, astrology, foot reflexology, voodoo and prayer, it's time for a visit to the drug store. You will find before you, a bewildering array of medications in various strengths and colors. (Don't laugh about the color; people have been found to respond to some colors of pills better than others, depending on the condition. Out of this mountain of pretty pills at the drug store, there are really only three basic types of pain-reliever: aspirin, acetaminophen and NSAIDS (nonsteroidal anti-inflammatory drugs.) The rest is a matter of dosage and hype. For minor pain, it makes little difference which type of pain reliever you use. Use the one you think works best for you. Tylenol is, in my opinion, an over rated pain reliever. It has none of the anti-inflammatory action of aspirin and is mediocre at best for pain relief. Not everyone agrees with that. Some swear by it. Who am I to argue?

According to pain expert Dr. Michael B. Jacobs, as pain becomes more intense, the NSAIDS (Advil, Nuprin, Motrin, Aleve) are more effective. I have my doubts about this. I remember the promotion of Darvon back in the 60s. It was "more effective" than aspirin or Tylenol and it was non-addictive and safe. <u>None of this turned out to be true</u> and Darvon has gone the way of bat manure in the treatment of pain. Ibuprofen, considered stronger than aspirin, may have the same fate as Darvon eventually. Some of the NSAIDs may cause serious kidney disease and there is evidence that they may affect fetal heart development.

For migraine headaches, Jacobs recommends a combination of aspirin and caffeine, such as Anacin. I suggest that Dr. Jacobs has never had a migraine headache because <u>none</u> of these compounds will do <u>anything</u> for a real migraine attack. Codeine or Demerol by mouth is quite effective if the migraine attack is caught early, especially Demerol. If the migraine attack is well established, you need a spheno-palatine ganglion block with cocaine solution. But you will not get it until you successfully promote a "freedom from pain" bill such as the legislation of California state Senator Green – see Appendix II.

Gall bladder attacks (Cholecystitis)— inflammation of the gall bladder which is located at the right upper quadrant of your belly, at the margin of your rib cage — are surprisingly amenable to home remedies. Hot compresses over the area of pain will often give quick relief. For reasons unknown, a thorough enema is also effective in relieving the pain of Cholecystitis. If you have had gall bladder attacks before and are thus familiar with the symptoms, this may be all the treatment you will need for this malady. It will probably recur and you will have to repeat the procedure outlined above. With the new endoscopic methods of surgery that are now available, surgical treatment of this disease is simpler, much safer and relatively painless. If you are having these painful attacks more often than twice a year, you should consider this surgery. An attack can become a dangerous emergency and so IT IS best to have it out.

Abdominal pain is a specialty in itself. If you procrastinate and self-medicate too long, the result can be disastrous. Appendicitis usually starts with pain in the right lower quadrant or with nausea. But the pain <u>may not</u> start at the right lower quadrant, as your appendix may be some where else. With physical examination and history, i.e., asking the patient some important questions, the diagnosis may be made by an astute doctor but, <u>even the best diagnostician</u> often will be wrong on this diagnosis. However, the British have invented a fiberoptic method of examination that seems to be <u>99 percent accurate</u>. They make a tiny incision in your abdomen and take a peek with a "medical telescope." This diagnostic procedure will save a lot of people an unnecessary operation and the subsequent pain – IF American surgeons will accept the procedure.

And there is more good news about appendicitis from British doctors. If the inflamed appendix is in the early stages of infection, a hefty dose of penicillin will arrest the condition and it seldom returns. Unfortunately, American surgeons aren't on to this, or simply don't accept it. They like to operate.

Eye pain — <u>don't fool around with pain in the eye ball</u>. See an ophthalmologist ASAP.

Joint pain — this covers a large field of pathology, from rheumatism, to gout, to fibromyalgia, to gonorrhea (surprise), to osteoarthritis, to German measles and other acute viral infections, to sickle cell anemia, to the bends, to rheumatic fever, to allergy, to porphyria and a dozen more diseases that I can't think of at the moment.

I always recommend first trying color therapy for joint pain. It is completely safe, simple and essentially costless. It may do nothing but it may be dramatic. <u>Stick with it</u> for at least a week. If the joint pain is severe, do it on a continual basis. For details, read *Color Me Healthy*, available from Rhino Publishing (www.rhinopublish.com).

On occasion, I have found neural therapy to be remarkably effective, especially where only one joint is involved. Neural therapy is the use of Procaine injections into the superficial layers of the skin around the inflamed joint. This is a German technique and when the reaction is near-miraculous, such as a complete clearing of a severely-inflamed joint in 24 hours, the German doctors call it a segunden -- "lightning reaction." I had one case like this and it astounded me.

A "non-working" class mother brought her son to me with Still's disease, rheumatoid arthritis of children. He had a severe, painful, rheumatoid right knee that could not be touched. He was terrified of doctors and the mother was extremely hostile, seeming to dare me to cure him. (I don't know why she brought him to me, desperation I guess. I knew the most I was going to get out of the case was a law suit — people don't realize how unpleasant it is to practice medicine these days. If the doctors all had a writing racket like me, or some other decent way to make a living, there wouldn't be any doctors left practicing medicine.)

So anyway, the child had a "lightning reaction" to the injection of the procaine into the skin around the knee joint. It took five of us to hold him down and I was deaf from the screaming for twelve hours. The mother called me the next morning. I answered with dread and started going through my Rolodex for the number of my attorney. "I have never seen anything like it," she said, "the knee is completely normal. I can't keep him still." No "thank you" or "the check's in the mail," or anything like that. <u>And I never heard from her again</u>. I can

think of only two explanations: (1) The rheuma-
tologist told her it was voodoo and a
coincidence or (2) If the Still's disease cleared
up completely on the therapy (and I don't think
it would have, but it might have) she would
then lose some state disability money and that
would be a very bad thing, worse than arthritis
from her point of view since <u>she</u> wasn't doing
the suffering. Am I overly cynical to think so
adversely of a mother? Maybe.

I didn't mean to spend so much time on neural therapy but it illustrates what's out there in
the way of alternatives and, besides, I thought
you would enjoy seeing how us doctors suffer.

Akin to neural therapy is Scar Therapy. Scar
therapy is related to the acupuncture meridians
and achieves remarkable results in some patients. My colleague, Milissa Tolifero, MD, who
practices in Arkansas, had a typical case in
which scar therapy brought about a reaction as
dramatic as the lightening reaction described
above in neural therapy.

There is a relationship between some scars
and nearby acupuncture points. As you may
know, acupuncture points don't have any relationship to parts of the body that make any
"sense." They are "conduction pathways" that
are unrelated in an anatomic sense to the conventional peripheral nerves. So a scar on the
forehead might cause chronic pain in the foot.
That's hypothetical as I don't know the actual

acupuncture points. But I <u>do</u> know that the injection of scars with procaine anesthetic can sometimes have remarkable results that you would not expect on a chronic pain site far removed from the scar.

FOR MEN ONLY

There is a common pain problem in men that is seldom discussed and is often misdiagnosed. Prostatodynia — pain at the pelvic floor, the perineum, which is the area between the penis and the anus.. The name indicates pain in the prostate but it may not be the prostate at all. The negative effect of Prostatodynia on men's lives can be profound. In surveys, it has been found to be at the level of heart attacks and angina in over all effect on life style. So it's obviously a pain that requires serious attention by doctors. Yet, the problem is "egregiously neglected," in pain research according to the journal, *Pain*. The authors of the article in *Pain* reported that they could find only two articles in this same journal over a period of <u>ten years</u> on the subject of perineal pain in men, Prostatodynia.

These unfortunate men receive all sorts of treatment from urologists, from surgery to drugs, usually with little or temporary results. But a remarkably simple treatment is available but little used. Harry C. Miller, the former chief of urology at George Washington University, recognized the prostate as a stress target just like the stomach--nausea, indigestion, heart burn and other symptoms under stress -- or the lungs with an asthma stress reaction.

Dr. Miller found that "stress management," i.e., explaining to the patient that overwork, fatigue, anxiety and other stress factors were responsible for the symptoms, which worked through the autonomic nervous system. He emphasizes to them that they do not have an incurable or transmissible infection and they do not have cancer or serious prostate disease. The knowledge that their symptoms were not a sign of serious disease but an <u>expected</u> physiologic response of the prostate to stress was remarkably potent therapy and resulted in 86 percent of the men treated reporting as being better, much better or cured. So here is an area of pain, not only from the condition itself but from the added pain of unnecessary surgery, that can be almost eliminated by common sense, understanding and patience.

The operation that probably produces the most unnecessary amount of pain in men is prostatectomy because the operation is so often unnecessary. The extirpation of the prostate was very much in vogue in the 19th Century. The brother of the author, Marcel Proust, Robert Proust, was a surgeon with a particular fondness for prostatectomies. He did so many of them that his colleagues referred to them as "Proustatectomies." The suffering was horrendous and, the way most surgeons treat pain, it's not that much better today. You want pain? I'll show you pain — let me give you a trans ure-thral resection (the Roto Rooter operation of the prostate through the penis). And you, being a big, brave boy, will want to dispense with that pain-relieving sissy stuff.

Akin to the agony of the "Proustatectomy" in the old days, was the probing of the bladder for stones in preparation for the <u>real</u> operation to come. (Women as well as men could enjoy this procedure.) Andre Pare', the father of modern surgery, listed the instruments to be employed in removing the stones: hooks, probes and duck-billed forceps. And how did the patient endure this nightmare sans anesthesia? His ankles were tied as were his hands. A rope around the neck secured his hands against his knees. Four men. "strong, not fearful and shy," held the patient securely and thus completed the surgical team. The operation, I suppose, was covered by the patient's health plan.

Dr. Pare' was not insensitive to the patient's suffering and he did his best to prepare the patient for the ordeal to come. He felt that the patient's attitude and inner strength was necessary for a successful outcome, even though he would have to be restrained by four men "strong, not fearful and shy."

Pare' respected the free will of his patients: "The indications as to the state of the patient's valor and strength must take precedence above all else for if he is failing or is in a weakened state, it is necessary to forsake all other things in order to be helpful to him as when necessity forces us to amputate a limb or to make some large incisions or other similar things. Nonetheless, because the patient does not have enough valor and strength to tolerate the pain, such operations need to be postponed (if possible) for long enough for nature to be restored and strength regained by good diet and rest." In the medicine of the time, the patient's cooperation and state of mind was considered indispensable to affect a cure.

SHINGLES AND POST-HERPETIC NEURALGIA

Shingles is a viral disease of the nerve endings manifested by grayish blisters on the skin surface. The lesions look like chickenpox and, in fact, it is a localized form of that childhood disease. They are not pretty and can be painful. But much worse is the neuralgia (nerve inflammation) that can persist after the original infection clears, usually in about two weeks. This is an extremely painful condition, post-herpetic neuralgia (PHN), can lead to suicide. There is no better example of pain neglect than PHN. It is a chronic condition. Therefore, the doctor reasons, pain-relieving narcotics must be used "judiciously." If the patient commits suicide, the doctor will not be blamed. The patient just didn't have the right stuff, and at least he didn't become a despicable narcotic addict -- better dead than drugged.

Spheno-palatine ganglion block is the treatment of choice and, if you can afford it, I would recommend that you seek out an ENT specialist in a foreign country who is competent at the procedure and where cocaine has not been banned for patient use (which is about anywhere but the USA). Neural therapy, described earlier, can be tried but the results are inconsistent.

Antiviral drugs are now being recommended. Oral acyclovir, if used early in the course of the acute stage, i.e., during the stage of the visible blisters of shingles, is said to reduce the incidence of PHN by 46 percent. That still leaves a lot of pain that needs narcotic relief.

Another neurological condition that is even more painful than PHN is trigeminal neuralgia — tic douloureux. This devastatingly painful condition causes facial pain along the route of the fifth cranial nerve, a sensory nerve that comes directly out of the base of the brain. The treatment of choice is, again, spheno palatine ganglion block with cocaine, one of God's greatest gifts to doctors for the treatment of suffering. But the Leviathan State is too busy chasing cocaine smugglers and users to concern itself with your little pain problem.

A new drug is being touted for the relief of trigeminal neuralgia pain. The drug is an anticonvulsant called gabapentin. Two cases have been tried and they had remained pain-free for six months at this writing. I would wait on this one. The pattern of therapy of this form of neuritis has been that of an immediate good response to a drug and then a gradual decrease in effectiveness — baclofen, phenytoin and carbamazepine have all eventually proven to be ineffective. Your best course is not to go to your doctor but to your congressman and urge support of a bill that will unshackle doctors and allow them to use what they need to relieve pain, including cocaine.

In the meantime, find a holistic doctor who will try neural therapy, scar therapy (if you have scars) and color therapy.

LEG CRAMPS

One of the most unpleasant and painful experiences of aging is "night cramps," a muscle spasm in the legs that occurs during the night or on awakening in the morning. The pain can be excruciating and can be relieved only by walking and vigorously massaging the affected muscle. It is more common in men. This has been a perplexing problem for doctors. Pain medication is of no avail because the cramp, with walking and massage, is gone before any medication can take effect. But it is a very unpleasant and painful experience, one that needs to be prevented rather than treated.

Fortunately, there is a treatment that works well in most cases. It is quinine sulfate, the drug used to prevent malaria in our troops in the early part of World War II. Quinine reduces the excitability of motor end-plates of skeletal muscles and thus prevents the cramps. But doctors are being frightened away from the use of quinine because of some overdose reports from the Scottish Medical Journal. An <u>overdose</u> of quinine sulfate, reported the journal, led to blindness in over ten percent of the 30 cases studied. Although this is irrelevant to the rational use of quinine, the proper dosage being small, many doctors are now afraid to use quinine for leg cramps! Note that this was an <u>overdose</u> report and had nothing to do with the rational use of the drug.

If you have never taken quinine, and so don't know if you are allergic to it, drink a bottle of quinine water in the morning before breakfast. If you experience allergy symptoms — itching, headache, runny nose or wheezing — you shouldn't take quinine. The tonic water taken at bedtime — six ounces — might be all that you need to suppress the cramps. If it isn't sufficient then you will need a prescription for quinine sulfate capsules.

PAIN IN THE LEGS ON WALKING ("Intermittent Claudication")

Let's call it IC to save space. IC is one of the poorest treated forms of agony in the devil's pantry of pain. It's caused by obstruction of the arteries of one or both legs. This blockage decreases the blood supply to the tissues and thus decreases the oxygen needed for exercise. When the patient attempts to walk, he gets "ischemic pain," from oxygen starvation of the muscles of the leg, usually the calf muscle.

The reason I say that IC is one of the poorest treated forms of pain is because there is a very effective therapy that doctors, especially the surgeons who want to operate on the legs, absolutely refuse to recognize and that's chelation therapy. <u>Chelation works</u> on intermittent claudication; it's proven beyond a doubt. And it's criminal that tens of thousands of patients suffer the pain and disability of this disease — until the surgeon cuts the leg off. Then he has a <u>different</u> pain — phantom limb, which is worse than IC.

The Chronic Pain Letter, which obviously devotes itself to pain, wrote a full page in their Vol. 14, #5 issue on a new concept for relieving the pain of IC. The procedure, called Spinal Cord Stimulation (SCS) appears to be quite effective in a high percentage of cases. But remember, this is only a symptomatic treatment and will not fix the cause of the pain – obstruction of the arteries in the leg. They make no mention of chelation therapy in this otherwise good article; it just isn't fashionable. I suspect that a combination of SCS and chelation therapy would give an immensely improved picture for this disease and would, for the most part, eliminate surgery for this condition.

SCIATICA

Sciatica, the lay term for sciatic neuritis, is perhaps not the King of Pain, but it's in the king's court, without a doubt. Dr. Eugene Lipov at the Poplar Creek Center for Pain Management, is now performing a new outpatient fiberoscopic medical procedure that could give relief to back pain sufferers without surgery. See appendix II for details on this promising treatment for a painful and debilitating condition.

MULTIPLE SCLEROSIS

This is one disease that deserves special mention because its particular discomforts and pains do not respond to the conventional opiates. This is not generally known, even by many doctors. A large-scale survey of more than 7,000 multiple sclerosis (MS) patients shows that most MS patients are under treated for pain. Even if they recognized the problem, most doctors would not know how to treat it because, for some bizarre neurological reasons, the pain of MS does not respond to the usual narcotics, such as Demerol, morphine and codeine. Neurologists use a combination of seemingly inappropriate drugs such as anticonvulsants and tranquilizers. No drug is uniformly successful.

SOME CONCLUSIONS

Doctors are being paralyzed into a state of uncertainty and uselessness sometimes brought

on by the patients. And the patients are confused. Many want an authoritarian figure for a
doctor who will tell them what to do and yet at
the same time, they are being told to "take control" of their treatment. They read a few
paperback books and then go to the doctor
armed with questions. They think they understand more than they do. The doctor is put in
the position of having to give a medical school
lecture on the patient's particular problem but
the patient does not have the scientific medical
background to really understand it. And the patients usually aren't willing to pay for the extra
time these discussions take. They'll pay a law-
yer by the hour but feel that the doctor's time
isn't as important — "All he did was give me a
prescription."

This has led to tremendous frustration and
resentment on both sides of the desk. The patients often demand too much and the doctors
often give too little. I don't know where it's all
going to end but a good start in the right direction would be for doctors to take pain relief
seriously. If doctors don't accept the responsibility of pain relief, they will lose what respect
they still have with the public.

When discussing pain and its relationship to
various organs, we could end up with a text
book. I have tried to cover major areas and major methods of treatment, both conventional and
"holistic." And I wanted to get across the con-

cept to you that your major enemy in the fight against the devil's diversion, pain, is under-treatment secondary to ignorance by doctors and "drug war" politics which paralyzes the doctor with fear.

There are a few rays of hope. A government report has actually urged new drug laws to protect patients from pain. It seems preposterous, as Otto Scott said, to have to entertain such legislation but that's the world in which we live. (Compass newsletter, www.the-compass.com) The government report is being released by the Institute of Medicine under the title "Approaching Death - Improving Care at the End of Life." The Institute of Medicine is a private organization of experts that provides medical policy advice under a congressional charter granted to the National Academy of Sciences. But don't count on this — government reports are just reports. If there is no pressure applied to the politicians, nothing will come of it.

Annals of Surgery, 1985;202:104-110
National Institutes of Health report on
    marijuana, 8/97
New England Journal of Medicine, 8/7/97
The Economist, 8/16/97
The New American, 13 October, 1997, pp35

THE NOVEMBER COALITION

EXPOSING THE FOLLY OF AMERICA'S WAR ON DRUGS

"We are a growing body of citizens whose lives have been gravely affected by our government's present drug policy. We are drug war prisoners, their loved ones, and others who believe that our present course of war in America has a price that we cannot afford to pay.

"Our goal is to make our voice heard, expose the folly of America's War on Drugs, and demand change. We are encouraged by the scores of Federal Judges, physicians, law enforcement officers, lawyers, mayors, governors, educators and legislators who have become outspoken critics of our country's current policy.

'"The statistics can get overwhelming: Over 70% of the 1.7 million American citizens currently behind bars are non-violent drug offenders. <u>The average sentence for a first time, non-violent drug offender is longer than that for a rapist, child molester, or bank robber</u>. This is insane and outrageous, but there's something about numbers: People don't get too worked up about them. But give people a human drama, and they'll go to the barricades. And no group has done more to put human faces on the statistics in our ongoing "War on Drugs" than the November Coalition.

"There is no question that the War on Drugs is fundamentally wrong in every way. Neither philosophically nor practically is there any rational justification for this ongoing travesty. But how often have you thought, really thought, about the individual victims? The first-time offenders whose lives are stolen from them; The spouses and children who are left behind to struggle on. Their stories are told here, and they are unforgettable.

"The cost is enormous and even some judges and DEA agents are speaking out against it. Over 70 percent of the people in jail today for non-violent crimes are offenders in drug possession or trafficking crimes. What is the cost? No one can say but it is in the tens of billions of dollars. Consider the cost of prison housing ($30 to $50 thousand a year per inmate), meals, guards, care for injuries, rapes, recreational facilities, "education," make work projects (which is involuntary solitude -- complain and you will be transferred to the living hell of a prison for murderers and the criminally insane). And who can say what the cost is to our culture -- disrespect for police and contempt for the law, broken homes and divorce, orphaned children. How can you measure that?

"At The Wall, the names, numbers, photos and stories of hundreds of prisoners are posted. You can flip through them, one by one. You will read about Cynthia Dickerson who was framed in a "reverse sting" by a pressuring "friend", and has a <u>9 year, 1 month, and 1 day</u> sentence to serve. (A judge would have to be a mentally ill, sadistic monster to hand out a strange sentence like that.) Terry Anderson, mother of 2, received a <u>30 year sentence</u> which is, in her words, "just one year shy of the length of time I've been on this earth.""

"The Children of War section is even more devastating. Read 10-year old Philip Gaines' letter to the judge, begging for his mother's freedom: "...my birthday is coming up in October the 25 and I need my mom to be here on the 25 and for the rest of my life." (The plea fell on deaf ears, and <u>first-time offender,</u> Dorothy Gaines, is serving a <u>19-year</u> sentence.)"

I urge you to support the November Coalition Foundation. Contact them at the following address:

The November Coalition Foundation, Inc.
795 South Cedar
Colville, WA 99114
(509) 684-1550
E-mail: <u>moreinfo@november.org</u> - -
Home Page: <u>http://www.november.org</u>

ACTION TO TAKE

I -- ON PATIENT SUFFERING

(1) If you have to have surgery, take this monograph to your surgeon and ask him if he has the courage to give you enough narcotic to avoid the hell of post-surgical pain, not just partially but nearly completely. This is perfectly feasible with modern pain-control technology with a surgeon who is up to date in these matters Most of them are not and <u>have never taken a course on pain management</u> — it's not cost effective.

(2) Ask your doctor to read the BMJ article reported above (British Medical Journal, 12/15/00). Call him the next day to see if he will use this safe procedure to enhance your comfort and increase the safety of the surgery. If he says no, get a second opinion.

(3) Work to have a bill passed in your state to free doctors from the dead hand of state and federal government — call it the Freedom from Pain bill. That label for your bill should catch the eye of a few million people in your state, or at least those who are in pain. Pattern it after the bill proposed by Senator Green of

California or after the New Jersey plan -- see below.

(4) New Jersey legislators take the pain issue so seriously that bills have been passed that will require health professionals to consider pain as a "fifth vital sign." This will force doctors to do their duty toward their patients in pain and perhaps shore up their courage in resisting the inhumane policies of the Washington drug "czars."

A second bill gets down to specifics: it provides patients with the "right to expect and receive appropriate pain assessment, management and treatment as integral components of their care."

Action to take:

Get similar bills passed in your state. (You're not getting any younger, you know – do you want to die in pain?) Write to NJ state senator Charlotte Vandervalk, thank her for her sterling work in the defense of patients' rights to freedom from pain, and ask her for copies of the following NJ laws: Assembly bill numbers 316, 317, 318 and 319.

(5) Buy in quantity copies of this book to promote your legislation. If you wish to copy it, we permit you to do so as long as you give the copies away and give our E mail address and Web site. Go for it! — the pain you save may be your own.

Ref: Pain Practice Management, Special Issue, 2000

II -- ON THE DRUG WAR

Read the book, *Our right to Drugs* by Thomas Szasz, MD. Dr. Szasz is a different type of psychiatrist -- he believes in the family and freedom. He recognizes that our enemy is the state. (See Appendix V for some excerpts from the Szasz book.) When I read a book, I always underline the important parts, in case I want to plagiarize it later. When I had finished, I realized I had underlined practically the whole book. <u>Don't be afraid to test your cherished beliefs on this issue</u>.

Dr. Szasz says: The mind boggles. We spend more money on medical care than any other people in the world. And what is the result? That we live in a society in which people who, according to doctors, should have no access to narcotics seemingly have unlimited (illegal) access to them, while people who, according to doctors, have the most urgent need for narcotics have little or no access to them. Who is at fault? No one. Everyone is a victim, including the physicians, who are concerned that they will lose their licenses or be prosecuted if they prescribe narcotics "in the amounts necessary to treat chronic severe cancer pain.

"The cancerous growth of....mendacious rhetoric now affects virtually every aspect of daily life. Thus, many types of self-medication are defined as diseases (and prohibited as crimes), while at the same time many persons defined as mental patients are routinely drugged against their will for their supposedly treatable alleged brain diseases."

Take the challenge and read this book. You'll still be the same person afterward; you'll still have your religious beliefs; you will still go to church on Friday, Saturday or Sunday. However, you will never feel the same about the war on drugs which is a war against private property, a war against privacy and a war to establish a <u>complete police state</u> run by crooks even worse than the ones we put up with now. (There are more quotes from the Szasz book in the Appendix of the hard copy edition but not the electronic edition due to copyright restrictions.)

We must erect an <u>Electronic Fence</u> at the Mexican border. This is the idea of Sam Cohen, the father of the neutron bomb. I have no idea what he is talking about, but I know if Dr. Cohen says it will work then I can assure you it would be (1) relatively inexpensive, (2) effective in keeping illegals out and (3) non-injurious. Sam is not getting any younger and so I hope he has given the basic scientific idea to someone to carry forward.

<u>Fortress America</u> -- If we get out of foreign wars, bring our troops home, quit aiding foreign countries and let them sink or fall on their own, we can rebuild our once-great nation and beat the drug problem. The Navy can protect our shores and the Army can protect our border

with Mexico with relative ease if an electronic fence is erected.

The ICBM threat isn't what it used to be and the government has no intention of protecting us from it anyway. A neutron radiation protection umbrella in space could shield the entire country, according to Sam Cohen. But no one will listen to him because anything to do with radiation for defense (or offense) is verboten. The American people are, through years of propaganda, paralyzed with fear on the radiation issue. I don't know why I got into the ICBM story here. The enemy wouldn't bombard us with drug-carrying missiles would they? Why should they? They are having great success by land, sea and air without using fancy space weapons.

Support the November Coalition.

Abolish the public schools. Is there anyone so blind as not to see that the public school system is at the heart of the problem? If you cannot afford a private school, preferably a religious one, then form a small association with your neighbors and home school, which is what you should have been doing in the first place.

Will some kids get left out? Of course they will. But they are better off with NO SCHOOLING than what they are getting now. It's not the state's business to improve the minds of your children. That's the last thing in the world they will ever accomplish. How did we get this <u>army of illiterates</u>, who went to state schools and now are roaming the streets? It's no stretch to say that <u>the public schools feed the drug problem</u>.

I discussed with a sophisticated investment banker in London the worldwide attack on those small countries trying to make a living providing confidential bank accounts.

There are two motives to this attack on the banking systems of small countries. They want to control their worldwide banking monopoly and they want control of tax revenues. Essentially, this amounts to control of the world. I ventured that the attack on the drug lords through the banking system was not productive. My banker friend replied, "No, it is <u>not</u> productive because the major dealers <u>now own their own banks</u>. What it amounts to, is a takeover of these small countries, an elimination of the competition, which had become too large to ignore. The billionaire drug dealers have nothing to fear. The corruption is too deep. If the fox owns the hen house, how can the hens be protected?"

SO WE MUST...

....<u>eliminate the federal drug "war" program</u> and divide the funds saved among the states. It should be a "states rights" issue but, as far as I can tell, no one has thought about it that way. At the state level, corruption is easier to identify and control. People don't care about drugs in foreign countries. They are more interested in saving Tuscaloosa than they are Tenerife, and saving Columbia, SC more than Columbia, South America. This is not a perfect solution; some states will do a better job than others. But if ANY of then do a good job it will be an improvement over the federal blunderbuss now in operation.

If the U.S. government refuses to back down on this self-destructive program -- and they are almost certain to refuse without massive rebellion among the people -- then we must take more drastic action. The next step would be...

Join "The Committee of 50 States," (C-50-S) based in Utah and chaired by J. Bracken Lee, the former governor of Utah. Their aim is to call for automatic secession by all the states if the national budget gets to $6 trillion. They should add to the program: or if the coke demand in the U.S. goes over $75 billion, or the total drug war budget goes over 20 percent of what it is at the inauguration of the C-50-S resolution, the 50 states will declare themselves independent. Then the states, as delineated above, could handle their own drug problems.

If 38 states cannot be persuaded to take the relatively moderate and bloodless secessionary action iterated in the last paragraph, then its time for the Patrick Henrys and the William Henry Lees to step forward and declare: "Whenever a government becomes destructive of these ends, it is the right of the people to alter or abolish it."

In case your history is a little rusty, that's from the Declaration of Independence.

So grab your pen and go to work "to alter or abolish" this unconscionable and oppressive dictatorship.

FINIS

APPENDIX I

THE CALIFORNIA STORY

California, for better or for worse, always leads the way in new political and social movements. This time it's for the better in that the legislature is trying to end the human suffering of patients in pain. It is not simple, the legislators found out to their dismay. Bureaucrats will simply keep doing what they are doing until challenged practically at gun point. An extreme example of this is the Clinton administration's disregard of rulings by the Supreme Court. The executive branch bureaucrats ignore all rulings not to their liking and ask: "How many troops does the Supreme Court have?"

We have gotten permission from the Journal, Sacramento Medicine, to publish the following report by Harvey L. Rose, M.D. :

In the fall of 1990, three events signaled a new era in the use of opioids for the management of chronic pain -- particularly non-malignant pain:

(1) SEDMS published "*The Painful Dilemma: The Use of Narcotics for the Treatment of Chronic Pain;*"

(2) Governor Deukmejian signed into law Senator Leroy Greene's SB 1802, the Intractable Pain Act, which protects physicians from unwarranted intrusion by regulatory agencies in the treatment of chronic pain with controlled substances. Under this law, a physician cannot be disciplined by the Medical Board for such treatment as long as a consultation was obtained from an appropriate specialist and good records were maintained on the patient;

(3) The AMA published "Balancing the Response to Prescription Drug Abuse," after becoming aware of the problem. As Dr. James Sammons stated, "The war on drugs should not be a war on patients." But it has been a war on patients and physicians alike.

In November 1990, my testimony was given before the Medical Board of California (MBC) and I asked them to communicate to the physicians of this state, through their Action Report, the significance of the year's prior events. Finally, in June 1991, the Action Report carried an article on the use of controlled substances for the management of chronic pain. While the article did mention Senator Greene's bill, no mention was made of "The Painful Dilemma" (Dr. Rose's article -- Ed..)

In October 1992, Senator Greene held hearings at the State Capitol regarding the Intractable Pain Treatment Act <u>because he was</u>

receiving calls from doctors informing him that
the regulatory climate had not improved at all.
At the hearing, physicians and patients testified
about the problems they encountered with prescribing and obtaining controlled substances for
chronic pain, but the Medical Board refused to
admit there was any problem.

On October 27, The Sacramento Bee reported "Legal Fears have Doctors Under-prescribing
Painkillers," and the following day Ken
Wagstaff resigned as director of the MBC over
an internal scandal. Governor Wilson subse-
quently appointed Dixon Arnett, a former
Republican assemblyman, to head the MBC.
Senator Greene, who knew Arnett from their
days in the legislature, met with him and expressed his concerns. Arnett, through friends
who had encountered difficulty getting medication for the relief of chronic pain, was aware of
the problem and set up a task force to look into
the situation. In its November 4, 1993 report, the
task force recognized that the under treatment
of chronic pain was a greater problem than
so-called "excessive prescribing."

After several hearings, the task force's statement on prescribing controlled substances for
chronic pain was published in the July 1994 Action Report (the guidelines are to be published
in an upcoming action report). In reference to
the report, Arnett was quoted in The Bee (8/11/
94), saying "Doctors won't have the Medical

Board to blame anymore (for under treatment of pain)." In addition, Arnett said in his letter to task force members that he wanted physicians to achieve a certain level of comfort when it comes to prescribing these drugs.

In November, Proposition 161, "Physician Assisted Suicide," appeared on the state ballot. A coalition of religious groups strongly opposed to the initiative spent large sums of money to defeat it, which they did, 54:46 percent. These groups came to realize that suicide was not the real issue at stake; rather, it was the pain. Cavalier and Associates, the same group that ran that campaign against Proposition 161 formed the California Pain Management Coalition. They worked with Assemblyman Richard Polanco, who introduced AB 2155 calling for a pain management advisory committee within the attorney general's office to advise on pain matters. The wife of an administrative assistant to Assemblyman Polanco had chronic pain and had experienced difficulty obtaining pain relief. Her doctors had been afraid of her getting "addicted" to opioids, but I maintain it was really the scarlet letter of "arrest" that kept her from getting what she needed to alleviate her pain.

AB 2155 passed that state legislature but was vetoed by Governor Wilson. In his veto message, however, the governor called for a pain summit to remove the impediments to adequate prescribing: "The proponents [of AB

21551] make a compelling argument that the medical community and the law enforcement community need to work together in a cooperative fashion to make certain patients are receiving medically necessary pain treatment. I am directing...the various boards...to overcome obstacles that contribute to inadequate pain management." 10/8/93

In 1989, the American Pain Society (APS) formed a new committee on analgesic regulatory issues. Ronald Blum, MD, chief of oncology at New York University, was the committee's first chairman. In 1987, <u>Dr. Blum had been arrested in his office by narcotic agents for alleged over pre-scribing of Diluadid to his cancer patients.</u>

They finally reduced the charges against him to not registering his patients as "narcotic addicts" as required by New York law. The second chair of this committee was Al Brady, MD, an oncologist from Portland, Oregon <u>who had also been arrested on charges similar to Dr. Blum's</u>. As a member of this committee, I worked with C. Stratton Hill, MD, head of oncology at MD Anderson Cancer Center in Houston. He was the author of The Intractable Pain Treatment Act, which had become law in Texas in 1989. We adopted this law, made a few changes, and it became law in California the next year. (Note that these arrested doctors are qualified specialists dealing in pain, yet they got "the scarlet letter of arrest." Under these insane conditions, what doctor who is not himself insane, would prescribe narcotics at all?)--Ed.)

William Marcus, deputy attorney general in the Los Angeles office, became a member of the APS's analgesic regulatory committee and gained awareness of how regulatory agencies had created a climate that was not conducive to prescribing narcotics for chronic pain patients.

The pain summit was held in Los Angeles in March 1994 with Senator Greene, as well as experts from all over the country in medicine, nursing, pharmaceutical manufacturing, and law enforcement, in attendance. At about the same time, the Agency for Health Care Policy Research came out with cancer pain guidelines, <u>acknowledging that at least half of all cancer patients are under treated for pain</u>. Certainly, addiction should not be an issue in deciding how much pain relief cancer patients can receive. The report on the pain summit, which was released in July 1994, stated that patients had a right to relief of their pain and suffering. The following was the only underlined statement in the summit report: "<u>We should create by statute a positive legal duty for physicians to relieve pain</u>." Included in the summit report was a chronology of events that had led up to the summit. The first event listed was Senator Greene's Intractable Pain Treatment Act.

In June, 1994, the 6th District Court of Appeals published a decision in the People vs.

Schade case. Among other charges, Dr. Schade was accused of illegally prescribing controlled substances to addicts (of course, these so-called addicts were actually chronic pain patients). Dr. Otto Neubuerger and I testified on Dr. Schade's behalf. One of the pivotal issues as seen by the court of appeals was the definition of addiction. In 1989, SB 711, another bill by Senator Greene, included a definition of addiction. It was passed by the legislature but vetoed by Governor Deukmejian.

The appellate court felt that if the trial court could not provide a definition of addiction, then how could it convict Dr. Schade for treating addicts? It overturned that part of Dr. Schade's conviction by 2:1. While the dissenting justice felt that Dr. Schade still should have been found guilty, he caught the essence of the problem in his opinion: "To be sure, there was abundant and divergent testimony during the course of this trial devoted to the meaning of addiction as that concept relates to pain management. It was apparent that the medical community is divided on the question of the appropriate use of narcotics for treatment of patients in chronic pain. One thing made clear by the expert testimony is that there is no commonly accepted medical standard by which to measure how much is too much to prescribe for any given patient presenting with the complaint of chronic pain. As appellant testified, each case will depend upon the doctor's assessment of the particular patient's level of comfort and ability of function." (Daily Appellate Report, 6/17/94:8291).

Part of my own testimony, quoted in the appellate courts decision, reads as follows: "Dr. Rose testified that he has prescribed narcotics to chronic pain patients with nonmalignant ailments. According to Dr. Rose, the quality of life is the bottom line and the doctor should be able to prescribe narcotics when necessary to restore function in the patients' lives." (Daily Appellate Report, 6/17/94:8275).

With the virtually simultaneous release of the Medical Board's task force statement and the governor's pain summit report this year, there is no turning back. Once the full implementation of these documents is realized, California will become the first political unit on the planet where the under treatment of pain and suffering will be considered illegal. All members of the health care team will have not only a professional obligation but a statutory positive legal duty to effectively relieve their patients' pain and suffering, and no longer will physicians have to tell their patients in pain to "just learn to live with it." (In the above report, underlining was added _ Ed.)

Ref: Sacramento medicine, November, 1994

APPENDIX II

NOTE: This is not the same procedure as the epidural anesthesia reported earlier. It is an improved form of spinal surgery to avoid much of the pain this type of surgery entails. (all underlining added)

A NEW PROCEDURE FOR PAIN STARTING IN THE BACK AND GOING DOWN THE LEGS ("SCIATICA") AND POSSIBLY FOR GENERAL BACK PAIN

The American Academy of Orthopedic Medicine estimates the total annual cost to society from low back pain is $100 billion, including $20 billion in direct patient medical bills. With the aging of the U.S. population, these numbers will only grow.

The FDA has approved the sale and distribution of a miniature fiberscope that allows physicians to explore the epidural space, which is the area surrounding the spine, with a surgical incision. Treating the spine in a minimally invasive manner is not a new idea. Dr. Michael Burman first investigated the use of endoscopes in the epidural space in 1931 when he removed eleven vertebral columns from cadavers and examined them using rigid urology endoscopes. He concluded that the procedure had tremendous potential, however, technology at the time did not make it practical.

The following list demonstrating some of the abnormal pathology that can be identified by epiduroscopy: scar tissues and adhesions, congenital hypoplasia of the blood vessels, tumors, hypertrophied ligamentum flavum, herniated nucleus pulposus, epidural cysts, and neuritis.

In the future, as this technology evolves, patients needing more aggressive therapeutic procedures such as laser neuroplasty, discectomy, and partial laminectomy may be able to be treated in the minimally invasive manner.

Dr. Richard Deyo, principal investigator for the U.S. Public Health Service, who headed up the Back Pain Outcome Assessment Team, states that most backaches are caused by soft tissues that do not show up on X-ray, CT scans, and MRI Studies at George Washington Medical Center concluded that CAT scans and MRI can be misleading. They performed MRI's on 67 people who had no history of low back pain and these studies showed bulging or degenerated discs in 35% of the younger patients and in essentially all of the older patients. These studies should lead practitioners to question why the majority of low back pain patients are routinely subjected to the expense of these imaging technologies when only 1-2% of this population are candidates for surgical intervention.

The purpose of epiduroscopy is to obtain a specific diagnosis of soft tissue pathology in the epidural space. Epiduroscopy provides a direct image of the anatomy of the epidural space in full-color and in real time. During epiduroscopy, physicians guide the stearable catheter to the area in question. Once in the general vicinity of the pain generator, the physician gently probes structures and asks the patient if the probing is replicating the pain that he is experiencing. By interacting with the patient, the physician can identify specific pathology that is causing pain.

Epiduroscopy is much more effective if the patient has not been operated on and it is used early in the course of diagnosis. Since epiduroscopy can diagnose soft tissue pathology in a minimally invasive manner, it makes sense to use epiduroscopy prior to any open surgical procedures.

Myelotec set out to develop miniature endoscopes with high resolution fiberoptic imaging bundles that were reasonably priced and disposable. The fragile nature and high cost of quality video imaging fibers made this impossible. Myelotec came up with a unique concept of utilizing a reusable fiberoptic system with a disposable catheter. The resulting product was a 2.6 mm disposable catheter with a two way steering mechanism, with a 1 mm scope channel, 1 mm working channel, and a .9 mm reusable optical system. Clinical investigations started in June of 1995 and over 200 patients have been treated to date.

"Epiduroscopy is a technological break-through that signals the beginning of a whole new era for the treatment of chronic back pain," the experts say.

Epiduroscopy is currently used for assisting in diagnostic procedures. As doctors become more familiar with directly visualizing spinal anatomy, many new treatments will evolve. In the future, the working channel can possibly be used with laser fibers to treat herniated discs in a minimally invasive manner. Physician creativity and training are the only obstacles to treating the majority of spinal pathology in a minimal invasive manner.

It appears the Epiduroscopy will evolve, as arthroscopy and laparoscopy did, to become the diagnostic and therapeutic instrument of choice for many procedures in the spine. Endoscopic procedures have proven to be safer, more effective, and less costly than open surgical procedures; the spine will not be an exception to the fact.

For more information, write to:
www.myelotec.com
Myelotec, 1800 McDonough Road, Suite 221, Hoffman Estates, Illinois 60192
Phone: (847) 608-6620 Fax: (847) 742-8495
Email: elipovmd@aol.com

APPENDIX III

Table 1: Reluctance to Prescribe Opioids for Chronic Pain

Questions	Agree (%)	Disagree (%)
Chronic pain of unknown cause should not be treated with narcotics even if this is the only way to obtain pain relief	22.8	66.3
It is appropriate to escalate a dose of narcotics above the usual range if the prognosis is less than 1 year.	77.2	10.6
If a chronic pain patient is active on the job, there is no possible justification for prescribing narcotics for pain.	10.7	79.7
Narcotics should be restricted to treatment of severe intractable pain.	30.5	64.4
Persons who fit the "profile" of a likely drug abuser should never be treated with narcotics.	26.1	65.5
Prognosis should be the primary factor in deciding whether a patient should receive opiates.	14.5	73.6
Patients who complain of pain out of proportion to its cause are usually drug abusers.	21.8	59.3
Using narcotics to relieve the pain of benign conditions is ill-advised.	31.5	57.5

Questions	Agree (%)	Disagree (%)
Even if patients have severe chronic pain, they should be treated with narcotics only when their illness has reached a terminal phase.	9.5	82.2
The presence of a physiologic basis for pain should be the primary factor when deciding to prescribe opiates.	42.6	41.4
I would never prescribe narcotics for a patient with chronic pain who is able to work.	8.8	79.1

Table 2: Questions Measuring Fear of Patient Addiction

Questions	Agree (%)	Disagree (%)
Any patient who is given narcotics for pain relief is at significant risk for addiction.	27.9	64.6
I would be extremely concerned about possible addiction if a member of my family were given morphine for chronic pain.	39.2	53.3
I must exercise caution when prescribing potentially addictive medications to patients with chronic pain.	92.8	5.1

Questions	Agree (%)	Disagree (%)
When narcotics are used to control chronic pain, addiction is a common outcome.	41.4	49.2
More than 5% of patients who receive narcotics for pain subsequently become addicts.	22.0	44.5

Table 3: Questions Measuring Fear of Drug Regulatory Agencies

Questions	Agree (%)	Disagree (%)
If I prescribe opiates for several months for a patient with chronic pain due to cancer, I am violating state law.	2.4	87.6
My colleagues are more willing to give narcotics for cancer pain than I am.	10.3	52.7
Prescribing narcotics for patients with chronic pain is likely to trigger a drug enforcement agency investigation.	26.4	59.4
Too many narcotic prescriptions lead to utilization reviews.	49.5	22.6
Pharmacists who receive several opiate prescriptions from a doctor are likely to report the doctor to a state review board.	22.6	44.8

Questions	Agree (%)	Disagree (%)
If I follow the same prescribing practices as other doctors in my field, I will not be investigated by a regulatory agency.	47.7	18.6
There are limits to the number of narcotics tablets a patient should be prescribed.	67.1	21.7
I give patients a limited supply of pain medications to avoid being investigated.	23.8	53.6

Table 4: Questions Measuring Knowledge About Pain and Pain Treatment

Questions	Agree (%)	Disagree (%)
Almost all chronic pain can be relieved with treatment. (True)	67.6	26.4
The majority of patients having chronic pain are under medicated. (True)	56.5	22.1
Psychologic dependence on narcotics very frequently results from legitimate prescriptions. (False)	53.9	37.3
Suicide with an overdose of narcotics prescribed for pain occurs very frequently. (False)	9.8	73.8
The best judge of pain intensity is the patient. (True)	79.3	14.0

Questions	Agree (%)	Disagree (%)
The health care provider is the best judge of pain intensity. (False)	13.2	76.1
Pain in a cancer patient is most likely due to treatment. (False) The tumor itself is most likely	3.9	84.0
the cause of pain in a cancer patient. (True)	67.0	21.5
Preexisting conditions not related to the cancer cause the most pain for cancer patient. (False)	7.6	65.3
Increasing requests for analgesics indicate unrelieved pain. (True)	54.1	30.7
Increasing requests for analgesics indicate tolerance to the analgesic. (False)	62.4	24.7
Almost all cancer patients suffer pain. (True)	53.9	30.7
Almost all cancer patients should receive opiates to relieve chronic pain. (True)	38.3	37.1

Table 5: Questions Measuring Psychologic Attributes Related to Pain and Pain Treatment

Questions	Agree (%)	Disagree (%)
Compliant patients are entitled to more of my time than noncompliant ones.	46.3	38.6
Those who contribute the most to society should get better health care.		
I do not like being referred patients with doubtful diagnoses.		
Life would be better if homosexuals and IV drug abusers were segregated into special groups.	16.3	65.8
If I knew that a prospective patient had an untreatable disease, I would avoid taking that patient if I could.	9.1	79.1
I resent tax money being spent on patients with self-inflicted diseases.	50.2	34.6
A doctor whose practice has few surprises has a lot to be grateful for.	34.7	42.9
It "bugs me" if a consultant I am working with after carefully reviewing a patient says, "I'm not sure."	8.3	73.6

Questions	Agree (%)	Disagree (%)
When laboratory reports give conflicting information, I get upset.	27.7	51.1
Conscientious patients deserve better health care than those with self-inflicted problems.	33.0	53.2
It bothers me when even a pathologist cannot find the cause of death.	35.3	41.5
More "health-care dollars" should be spent on those who contribute most to society.	26.2	55.5
I do not enjoy treating patients whose illness is unlikely to respond to treatment.	50.7	37.7
I get irritated by inconsistent medical reports.	41.7	34.7
When the time comes that medical care will have to be rationed, those with high IQs should get the best care.	4.1	81.4
I dislike having patients whose outcomes "don't follow the book."	19.7	52.1
Undiagnosable illnesses are something I'd rather not get involved with.	31.9	47.7

Table 6: Questions Measuring Bias About Sex and Age

Questions	Agree (%)	Disagree (%)
It is easier for a male patient to become addicted to narcotics than a female.	3.8	65.0
Men are less likely to report pain to their doctor than women.	47.8	32.7
Females are more likely to experience pain than males.	23.0	45.0
Young adults are more likely to become addicted to narcotics than the elderly.	24.1	48.4
Older patients are less likely to report pain than younger patients.	30.9	38.6

APPENDIX IV

The War on Drugs: An Impossible Dream

Remarks By Senior Judge John L. Kane
of the U.S. District Court of Denver,
Colorado

Presented to the Western Governors'
Association in Scottsdale, Arizona on
December 15, 2000

The heedless pursuit of folly is a condition of human nature that has been with us throughout the history of mankind. With a collective refusal to recognize the inevitable and the obvious, various societies have thrust themselves headlong toward failure and disaster. The horror of the Children's Crusade is easy to admit because time has made it remote. A nation half-slave and half-free marching inexorably to Civil War is closer in time and consequence, but memory dims the barbarity and conceals fratricide in illusions of glory. Only recently have we dared admit the cultural ignorance and rejection of previous military counsel that were responsible for the national disaster we call Vietnam.

A monster gnawing in the belly of the human spirit impels us to abandon both cherished values and common sense. Like Don Quixote we depart from reality to pursue imagined demons and leave naught but carnage and confusion behind. The sated monster laughs at our folly and awaits the next imagined peril.

As Mark Twain observed, "What you know that isn't true will cause you more harm than what you don't know at all."* What we know that isn't true and what we refuse to know that is true about drugs forms the bedrock of our current national, indeed international, folly.

It is not true that illegal drug use is the nation's most serious health problem. Voluntary obesity is. More death and economic loss are caused by the consumption of legal drugs, principally alcohol and tobacco, than all illegal drugs. Over 100 million Americans drank alcohol last month. Over 50 million smoked tobacco. Nine million Americans smoked marijuana last month, 1.2 million ingested cocaine during the same period and fewer than 6 million used it within the past year. The figures for heroin and nonprescribed amphetamine abuse are so small they are not even in the same statistical league, much less the same ballpark.

Not all people who drink alcohol or smoke tobacco are killed or seriously injured as a result, nor are all voluntarily obese people fatalities. The same is true of those who take illegal drugs: not all, nor even most who use them are killed, seriously injured or addicted. Yet it is our stated national policy to imprison all those who possess, sell or use illegal drugs. That policy is pure folly.

Drug prohibition doesn't work. In 1914 when drugs like cocaine were available on grocery shelves, 1.3% of the population was addicted. In 1979, before the so-called "War on Drugs" crackdown, the addiction rate was still 1.3%. Today, while billions of dollars are being spent to reduce drug use, the addiction rate is still 1.3%. Yet America imprisons 100,000 more persons for drug offenses than the entire European Union imprisons for all offenses. The European Union has 100 million more citizens than the U.S.

Drug prohibition is also a waste of money. Local, state and federal governments now spend over $9 billion per year to imprison 458,131 drug offenders. Incarcerating all cocaine users for a year would cost $74 billion, but only after constructing 3.5 million more prison beds at an initial cost of $175 billion. It would cost $365 billion to jail everyone who smoked marijuana last year – five times the total state and local spending for all police, courts and prisons. We would need a cadre of guards and other prison employees larger than all of our military forces. This is a cost we cannot afford and a project we could never accomplish even if we had the money.

More costly than money, however, is the price we pay for this failed policy in terms of the decline in public safety, the breakdown of our criminal justice system, the erosion of our civil liberties and the pervasive public disrespect of the law.

Good citizens, who are otherwise law-abiding, ignore or evade drug laws. With literally tens of millions of people using illegal drugs or related to those who do, a large portion of the population has become cynical about all laws and our legal system and political process in particular.

Much like in the days of Prohibition, when citizens, politicians, children and gangsters met on common ground in speakeasies and paddy wagons and when judges and prosecutors sought the flimsiest of reasons to dismiss cases against the franchised populace, ordinary people today transact purchases with criminals in the black market. Hostility and scorn toward law and law enforcement are a natural consequence. When approximately half of the members of a high school graduating class have smoked marijuana or snorted cocaine, few, if any, of them or their parents are willing to regard them as criminals. Each year since 1989, more people have been sent to prison for drug offenses than for violent crimes. At the same time only one in five burglaries is reported and only one in 20 reported burglaries ends in arrest and yet detectives continue to be reassigned from burglary details to investigation of street sales of drugs.

On an even more practical level, the War on Drugs is doomed to failure. The most fundamental concept of economics is the law of demand, which says that consumers buy less when the price rises. Misunderstanding this basic rule, the drug warriors attempt to justify interdiction. They claim drug consumption can be ended by cutting off supply, thereby causing a price increase resulting in little or no demand. In other words, interdiction will cause prices to rise to such a high level that demand will cease.

A little knowledge is very dangerous. In fact, the law of demand only applies to one product at a time. Our sorry experience shows that when one illicit commodity becomes too expensive, another is selected. A 1994 National Bureau of Economic Research study found that when the price of marijuana rises, youth drink more beer and that directly correlates with an increase in traffic fatalities.

A National Institute of Justice study reported a precipitous increase in the use of methamphetamine during 1985-86 after a crop destruction program eviscerated the marijuana supply in Hawaii. Making marijuana more difficult to obtain also causes an increase in cocaine consumption. When efforts to interdict marijuana are successful, the danger to our youth is increased by a rising consumption of alcohol and cocaine. When the supply of beer is reduced, the consumption of hard liquor increases.

Moreover, interdiction increases production and consumption of drugs. A 1992 United States House Judiciary Crime Subcommittee reported that the massive effort to destroy the Medellin Cartel resulted in an increase of cocaine trans-shipment points from 11 to 25 and an expansion of cocaine processing to as many as 13 more countries. Researchers have also found a statistically significant correlation between higher incarceration rates of drug offenders and greater, not less, drug use.

As Benson and Rasmussen observe, the failure of the War on Drugs makes legalization an attractive alternative in the eyes of conservative and liberal luminaries such as esteemed Nobel Laureate Milton Friedman; author and commentator William F. Buckley, and former Secretary of State George Shultz on the one side, and former Baltimore Mayor Kurt Schmoke, New York Times columnist Anthony Lewis and ACLU President Nadine Strossen on the other. They all publicly advocate legalization of drugs, treating them like alcohol and subjecting them to advertising restrictions, age limits, time and place restrictions and excise taxes. For many, legalization is the logical solution to the nation's drug problems. For some, it is not only logical, but a matter of fundamental freedom. People are responsible for themselves and should have the right to make their own decisions.

Prohibition has always failed and always will, but there is an alternative to outright legalization. We are not forced to make a Hobson's Choice. The drug problem will evaporate when the black market is eliminated, but the evaporation process will take time and effort.

The middle approach between the extremes of legalization and prohibition is to accept drug use as an undesirable part of the human condition and treat it as a health problem. A 1994 Rand study shows that treatment of heavy cocaine users is seven times more effective than asset forfeitures, arrest and imprisonment. The same study shows that the cost of treatment is one-fourth that of police enforcement.

As Americans, our biggest fault is the overriding desire to solve any problem, "once and for all." To borrow from drug culture vernacular, our national psyche demands a "quick fix." Unfortunately, it isn't there. What we as a nation must do is learn to live with uncertainty and expect less than total success.

If our appraisal of American history is honest, we must recognize that our country has succeeded when it has placed its faith and trust in the spirit of American enterprise and that we have failed when we have followed a puritanical path. Our highest purposes are achieved when we proceed with the consent of the governed. Our failures occur with force, the threat of force and the practice of fraud. American drug policy includes the use of military force in other countries and on our national borders, the threat of force to other nations, and the threat of severe economic and diplomatic sanctions even to long-standing allies. In furtherance of that policy, the dissemination of false and misleading data by the government has become commonplace. The same policy results in ignoring, deriding and distorting facts that would otherwise show more successful alternatives to the present practices of interdiction and criminal sanctions for drug consumption.

Police agencies still need to protect the public by holding those who cause accidents or commit crimes while under the influence of drugs and alcohol fully accountable for their acts, but we must get them out of the business of financing their operations through the seizure and forfeiture of private property. The costs of law enforcement should be funded from the public fund under direct legislative control. In other and harsher words, we need to terminate the symbiotic business relationship that law enforcement has with the illegal drug industry. Each scratches the other's back.

One of the longest and most cherished traditions of this nation is that the military is subservient to the civilian government, and that military might shall never be engaged in domestic matters. <u>For as long as we have been free, we have disavowed the existence of a national police force. Law enforcement is the business of local police agencies. Federal grants and financing of multi-governmental task forces coupled with military assistance seriously jeopardize local control of police action. The federal government must get out of domestic drug law enforcement for no reason less important than the freedom of all individuals</u>.

State and local officials are responsible for domestic law and order. There is an understandable temptation for state officials to shape their policies and programs to conform to federal grant requirements, but state legislatures must insure that control of state agencies is not abdicated in the grab for federal funds. Indeed, if legislators do not meet this responsibility, they can be defeated at the polls and replaced by those who will. Community safety and freedom must not be compromised in pursuit of the federal dollar

Alexis de Tocqueville called our states and communities the "laboratories of democracy," where experiments in self-government could take place and the success of one could be substituted for the failure of another. <u>Our federally</u>

directed drug control policy has closed these laboratories. The consequence is that as a free people we continue to pursue but one path – the path of folly.

In order to deal successfully with drug abuse, this nation must eliminate the black market and permit a regulated one. We must permit the several states to resume their role as laboratories of democracy in which policies and programs suitable to their individual needs and conditions can be implemented. We must restore local authority and autonomy over police practices. Most importantly, we must confront drug abuse as a threat to health treatable through science rather than superstition and hysteria.

(underlining added)

APPENDIX V

THE WISDOM OF DR THOMAS SZASZ

The following quotes from **Our Right to Drugs** by Thomas Szasz, MD, Copyright ©1992, are reprinted with the kind permission of the publisher, Greenwood Publishing Group, Inc., Westport CT.

We sincerely hope that you will buy this book in quantity and give them to people you care about. It is a very powerful weapon for sanity in this period of madness and police state oppression, both domestically and internationally. [Underlining added by this author.]

We have launched ourselves on a self-contradictory quest for a veritable medical dystopia, that is, for an America free of drug abuse because doctors effectively control drug use, and where everyone dies a painless and pleasant death because benevolent doctors kill "dying" people who want to be killed. My point is that - having combined a dread of dying a protracted, pointless, and perhaps painful death with a fear of living with a free market in drugs - we have negated our chances for attaining pharmacological autonomy, that is, freedom vis-a-vis drugs similar to the freedom we enjoy vis-a-vis food or religion. Deprived of drugs useful for committing suicide, we nevertheless continue to cling to the hope of receiving the drugs we need to die a painless death when we are terminally ill The result is that we now seriously entertain the preposterous idea of giving doctors and judges the right to kill us. In view of our faulty premises, the appalling conclusion that "medical euthanasia" is preferable to a free market in drugs is quite logical: We abhor and reject the idea of granting adults legally unrestricted access to drugs suitable for suicide; we view the desire to die as a symptom of mental illness; we interpret virtually all suicide as a tragedy that ought to have been prevented; and we forget that euthanasia, mercifully administered by "ethical" doctors, is a particularly sinister gift totalitarian governments have bestowed on modern man. In short, I believe that one of the main reasons we reject a free market in drugs is because we fear having an unfettered opportunity to kill ourselves (which a free market in drugs necessarily entails) and expect a grand alliance between medicine and the state to solve our existential tasks of living and dying for us.

The mind boggles. We spend more money on medical care than any other people in the world. And what is the result? That we live in a

society in which people who, according to doctors, should have no access to narcotics
seemingly have unlimited (illegal) access to
them, while people who, according to doctors,
have the most urgent need for narcotics have little or no access to them. Who is at fault? No one.
Everyone is a victim, including the physicians,
who are concerned that they will lose their licenses or be prosecuted if they prescribe narcotics
"in the amounts necessary to treat chronic severe
cancer pain." Sydenham, as I noted at the beginning of this chapter, attributed the miraculous
powers of opium to relieve pain and suffering to
the Almighty God. What God has given, the
therapeutic state has taken away.

####

"Prescribing old psychoactive drugs such as
the barbiturates has thus become tantamount to
medical malpractice, whereas prescribing new
psychoactive drugs such as Prozac is viewed as
the hallmark of practicing scientific medicine.
The newer the drug the better, as the story of
Prozac illustrates. Launched in 1988 by Eli Lilly
and Company, Prozac was hailed for helping "to
revolutionize the treatment of depression by
stressing the biochemical nature of the disorder." Sales for 1989 were approximately $600
million, up 65 percent from 1988. In 1992, sales
of Prozac are expected to exceed $1 billion. I be-

lieve Prozac is so popular with patients and doctors alike not because it is therapeutically effective (what is the disease being treated?), but rather because most people like the way the drug makes them feel and because - it not being a controlled substance-doctors feel secure prescribing it. Moreover, the manufacturer is so eager to encourage the use of Prozac that it has done something unprecedented in the history of promoting so-called ethical (prescription) drugs: It has sent letters to physicians, promising to "defend, indemnify, and hold you harmless against claims, liabilities or expenses arising from personal injury alleged to have been caused by Prozac."

Nevertheless, most Americans support the War on Drugs, confirming Randolph Bourne's insight that "war is the health of the State, It automatically sets in motion throughout society those forces for uniformity, for passionate cooperation with the Government in coercing into obedience the minority groups and individuals which lack the larger herd sense."

"...it is difficult to escape the conclusion that, notwithstanding the contrary evidence of impressive scientific and technological achievements, we stand once again knee-deep in a popular delusion and crowd madness: the Great American Drug craze."

****

"Blind to the implications of interpreting in-temperance as illness, drug prohibitionists complain that drug addicts and alcoholics "qualify as disabled...(and that) the federal government is paying some $1.4 billion annually to 250,000 substance abusers -- who often spend the money on the substance, not on treatment."

The calculated use of the word "treatment," in lieu of the word "punishment," has long been the stock-in-trade of lawyers, politicians, and mental health professionals."

****

"The cancerous growth of this mendacious rhetoric now affects virtually every aspect of daily life. Thus, many types of self-medication are defined as diseases (and prohibited as crimes), while at the same time many persons defined as mental patients are routinely drugged against their will for their supposedly treatable alleged brain diseases.

"...we must keep in mind that the psychiatrist's evaluation of the effectiveness of such 'treatments' is misleading, to put it mildly. Somatic interventions imposed on involuntary mental patients authenticate the psychiatrist's precarious medical identity. Not surprisingly, the history of psychiatry is replete with instances of psychiatrists embracing various somatic interventions -- from bloodletting to lo-botomy -- as effective treatments. In short order, every one of these interventions proved to be worthless, or worse. I predict that the same fate will befall the use of so-called antipsychotic drugs. The evidence is already compelling."

****

"Drug prohibitionists often justify their poli-cies by claiming that the drug abuser's addiction spreads from using a "gateway drug" such as marijuana to using "hard drugs" such as heroin and crack. I doubt it. There is evidence, however, that the drug law-abuser's addiction spreads from using the coercive apparatus of the state to control recreational drugs, to using it to control recreational foods, and much else besides. Kelly D. Brownell, a professor of psy-chology at Yale, seriously suggests putting "a surcharge on foods with high fat and low nutri-tional value...the true battle must be waged against an increasingly seductive environment." Note that Brownell blames the choice to ingest more calories than one burns not on the failure of a particular actor to resist the temptation to overeat (or on his other personal reasons for be-having as he does), but on the "seductive environment" in which he is forced to live -- in short on our being blessed with an abundance of affordable good food."

****

"Nearly everything the American government, American law, American medicine, the American media, and the majority of the American people now think and do about drugs is a colossal and costly mistake, injurious to innocent Americans and foreigners, and self-destructive to the nation itself."

****

"We do not blame the obesity of fat persons on the people who sell them food, but we do blame the drug habits of addicts on the people who sell them drugs."

****

"Freud's anti-capitalist remarks were not isolated comments, tossed off at the spur of the moment. Years before, he greeted the Bolsheviks' declaration of war on private property and religious freedom with a mixture of naiveté and optimism. 'At a time when the great nations announce that they expect salvation only from the maintenance of Christian piety,' he wrote in 1917, 'the revolution in Russia--in spite of all its disagreeable details--seems none the less like the message of a better future.'

"The pathetic and now discredited principles of statist -- that is, Soviet -- economics thus continue to flourish in our own drug-control and mental-health systems."

****

"Sadly, the very concept of a closure of the free market in drugs is likely to ring vague and abstract to most people today. But the personal and social consequences of a policy based on such a concept are anything but abstract or vague, Every aspect of our life that brings us into contact with the manufacture, sale, or use of substances of pharmacological interest of people has been utterly corrupted.

"The result is that, in all the complex human situations we call "drug abuse' and "drug abuse treatment," the voluntary coming together of honest and responsible citizens trading with one another in mutual trust and respect has been replaced by the deceitful and coercive manipulation of infantilized people by corrupt and paternalistic authorities, and vice versa, the principal role of medical, and especially psychiatric, professionals in the administration and enforcement of this system of chemical statism is to act as double agents - helping politicians to impose their will on the people by defining self-medication as a disease, and helping the people to bear their privations by supplying them with drugs. <u>This is a major national tragedy whose very existence has so far remained unrecognized</u>."

****

"The War on Drugs has many grave consequences. In this discussion I can touch on only a

few of them. Perhaps the most obvious consequences of drug prohibition are the explosive
increase in crimes against persons and property
and the corresponding increase in our prison
population. Both phenomena are typically attributed to 'drugs,' a misleading locution for
which the media bears and especially heavy responsibility."

****

"I shall not belabor the fact that drugs do
not, indeed cannot, cause crime. Suffice it to repeat that crime is an act; that the criminal actor,
like all actors, has motives; and that drug prohibition provides powerful economic incentives
for both the trade in prohibited drugs and
crimes against persons and property."

****

"In 1884, protesting the arguments of (alcohol) prohibitionists, Dio Lewis -- a physician and
temperance reformer -- declared, 'Every man has
a right to eat and drink, dress and exercise as he
pleases. I do not mean moral right, but legal
right.' The profound truth of this simple statement is reflected, I believe, in an important
inference that we ought to -- but never do -- draw
from the Prohibition Amendment.

"The men who drafted the Volstead Act,
which provided for enforcement of the Eight-
eenth Amendment, wanted to prohibit the
consumption of alcohol; however, they did not

outlaw it. They were not interested in whether people transported bottles of chemicals from one place to another, yet that is what they outlawed. I infer from this that, deep in their hearts, they and their constituents realized that a competent adult in the Land of the Free has an inalienable right to ingest whatever he wants. It should be unnecessary to add (but our current drug scapegoating justifies my adding) that <u>there was no question, during Prohibition, of randomly testing people to determine if there was any ethanol in their system, or of searching their homes for alcohol, or of imprisoning them for possessing alcohol, or of involuntarily treating them for the disease of unsanctioned alcohol use</u>.

****

"Drug prohibitionists thus proudly proclaim that protecting people from themselves is just as legitimate a goal for criminal as well as civil law as protecting people from others. Accordingly, trying to save people from their own drug-using proclivities is considered to be ample warrant for depriving individuals of life, liberty, property, and any or all constitutional protections that obstruct this lofty goal."

****

"Why did a majority of the U.S. Supreme Court hold, as recently as 1911, that not only is selling cocaine, heroin, and other "dangerous drugs' a constitutionally protected right, but so is making false claims about their therapeutic efficacy? Because the Court presumably believed that property rights and personal rights cannot endure without a marketplace governed by the principle of caveat emptor. According to this principle, the government is required to protect buyers only from products that are mislabeled in the sense that the contents are falsely identified. If a person wants to buy a bottle of aspirin, the government must protect him from vendors who might sell him a bottle labeled 'aspirin' but containing arsenic.

"By the same token, this principle requires the government to leave the buyer alone to make his own decision. If you claim that vitamin C cures cancer of the common cold, and if I choose to believe you and want to buy vitamin C, I ought to be left free by the government to believe or disbelieve you and act accordingly. <u>It is not the duty of the drug manufacturer, the pharmacist, the physician, or the state to protect people from the consequences of acting on false beliefs. If it were, where would that leave religions and those who teach religious beliefs</u>?

****

[Quoting Mark Twain] "There are people who strictly deprive themselves of each and every eatable, drinkable and smokable which has in any way acquired a shady reputation. They pay this price for health. And health is all they get. How strange it is!" Dr. Szasz added: "Mark Twain did not live long enough to see something even stranger, namely, the American government's resorting to the use of naked force to impose this idea on people…"

REFERENCES

Freedom Daily
> Nov., 1996
> Tel.: (703) 934-6101 — $18 a year,

Privacy Alert (highly recommended)
> Vin Supryonwicz, editor
> privacyalert@thespiritof76.com
> Monthly -- $96 per year

Compass **newsletter**, 1/96
> Uncommon Media
> P.O. Box 69006, Seattle, WA 98168
> 12 monthly issues, $50.
> A unique newsletter for the conservative, intellectual reader — enthusiastically recommended.

A History of Pain, Roselyn Rey, Harvard University Press

Our Right to Drugs, Thomas Szasz, MD, Syracuse University Press

Chronic Pain Letter, Vol. XIV, #3, 1997

The Pill Book Guide to Over-The-Counter Medications
> Bantam Books, $6.99

Pain, 1995; 62:251

Lancet, 1996; 348:138

Archives of Internal Medicine, 1997;157:909-912

Scottish Medical Journal, 1997;42:8-9

THE CHALLENGE OF PAIN. Revised edition. Ronald Melzack and Patrick Wall, Penguin USA, 1989.

SCIENTIFIC AMERICAN, Ronald Melzack February 1990 Volume 262 Number 2

TEXTBOOK OF PAIN. Second edition. Edited by Patrick D. Wall and Ronald Melzack., Churchill Livingstone, Inc., 1989.

Journal of Pain and Symptom Management, Vol. 4, No. 3, pages 112-116; September, 1989.

Associated Press, 9/18/97

Neurology, 1997;48:1467

Journal of Pain and Symptom Management, 1995;10:265-266

Pain digest, 1996;6:143-144

Orlando Sentinel, 9/24/97

Chronic Pain Letter, Vol. XIV, #5, 1997

American Journal of Surgery, 1985;149;397-402

Journal of Pain Symptom Management, 1997;13:254-261.

New York State Journal of Medicine, 1976; 76:366-368

British Journal of Surgery, 1992;6:101-105

Pain Digest, 1997;7:200-203

Journal of Vascular Surgery, 1990;12:354-360

Annals of Surgery, 1985;202:104-110

National Institutes of Health report on marijuana, 8/97

New England Journal of Medicine, 8/7/97

The Economist, 8/16/97

The New American, 13 October, 1997, pp35

****

About Doctor William Campbell Douglass II

Dr. Douglass reveals medical truths, and deceptions, often at risk of being labeled heretical. He is consumed by a passion for living a long healthy life, and wants his readers to share that passion. Their health and well-being comes first. He is anti-dogmatic, and unwavering in his dedication to improve the quality of life of his readers. He has been called "the conscience of modern medicine," a "medical maverick," and has been voted "Doctor of the Year" by the National Health Federation. His medical experiences are far reaching-from battling malaria in Central America - to fighting deadly epidemics at his own health clinic in Africa - to flying with U.S. Navy crews as a flight surgeon - to working for 10 years in emergency medicine here in the States. These learning experiences, not to mention his keen storytelling ability and wit, make Dr. Douglass' newsletters (Daily Dose and Real Health) and books uniquely interesting and fun to read. He shares his no-frills, no-bull approach to health care, often amazing his readers by telling them to ignore many widely-hyped good-health practices (like staying away from red meat, avoiding coffee, and eating like a bird), and start living again by eating REAL food, taking some inexpensive supplements, and doing the pleasurable things that make life livable. Readers get all this, plus they learn how to burn fat, prevent cancer, boost libido, and so much more. And, Dr. Douglass is not afraid to challenge the latest studies that come out, and share the real story with his readers. Dr. William C. Douglass has led a colorful, rebellious, and crusading life. Not many physicians would dare put their professional reputations on the line as many times as this courageous healer has. A vocal opponent of "business-as-usual" medicine, Dr. Douglass has championed patients' rights and physician commitment to wellness throughout his career. This dedicated physician has repeatedly gone far beyond the call of duty in his work to spread the truth about alternative therapies. For a full year, he endured economic and physical hardship to work with physicians at the Pasteur Institute in St. Petersburg, Russia, where advanced research on photoluminescence was being conducted. Dr. Douglass comes from a distinguished family of physicians. He is the fourth generation Douglass to practice medicine, and his son is also a physician. Dr. Douglass graduated from the University of Rochester, the Miami School of Medicine, and the Naval School of Aviation and Space Medicine.

You want to protect those you love from the health dangers the authorities aren't telling you about, and learn the incredible cures that they've scorned and ignored?
Subscribe to the free Daily Dose updates "...the straight scoop about health, medicine, and politics." by sending an e-mail to real_sub@agoramail.net with the word "subscribe" in the subject line.

Dr. William Campbell Douglass'
Real Health:

Had Enough?

Enough turkey burgers and sprouts?

Enough forcing gallons of water down your throat?

Enough exercising until you can barely breathe?

Before you give up everything just because "everyone" says it's healthy...

Learn the facts from Dr. William Campbell Douglass, medicine's most acclaimed myth-buster. In every issue of Dr. Douglass' Real Health newsletter, you'll learn shocking truths about "junk medicine" and how to stay healthy while eating eggs, meat and other foods you love.

With the tips you'll receive from Real Health, you'll see your doctor less, spend a lot less money and be happier and healthier while you're at it. The road to Real Health is actually easier, cheaper and more pleasant than you dared to dream.

Subscribe to Real Health today by calling 1-800-981-7162 or visit the Real Health web site at www.realhealthnews.com.
Use promotional code : DRHBDZZZ

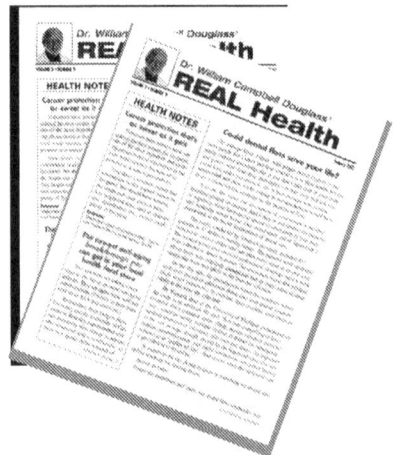

If you knew of a procedure that could save thousands, maybe millions, of people dying from AIDS, cancer, and other dreaded killers....

Would you cover it up?

It's unthinkable that what could be the best solution ever to stopping the world's killer diseases is being ignored, scorned, and rejected. But that is exactly what's happening right now.

The procedure is called "photoluminescence". It's a thoroughly tested, proven therapy that uses the healing power of the light to perform almost miraculous cures.

This remarkable treatment works its incredible cures by stimulating the body's own immune responses. That's why it cures so many ailments--and why it's been especially effective against AIDS! Yet, 50 years ago, it virtually disappeared from the halls of medicine.

Why has this incredible cure been ignored by the medical authorities of this country? You'll find the shocking answer here in the pages of this new edition of Into the Light. Now available with the blood irradiation Instrument Diagram and a complete set of instructions for building your own "Treatment Device". Also includes details on how to use this unique medical instrument.

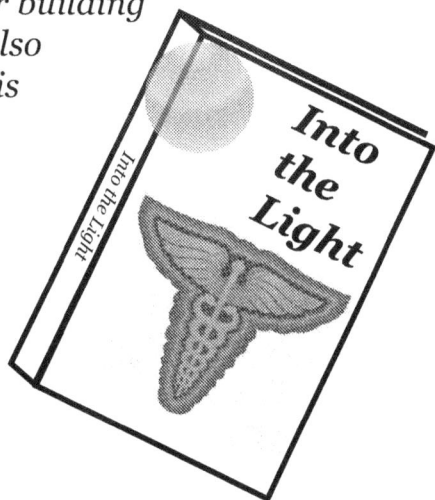

Into the Light

Into the Light

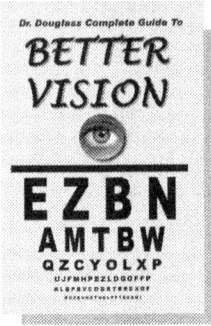

Dr. Douglass' Complete Guide to Better Vision

A report about eyesight and what can be done to improve it naturally. But I've also included information about how the eye works, brief descriptions of various common eye conditions, traditional remedies to eye problems, and a few simple suggestions that may help you maintain your eyesight for years to come.
-William Campbell Douglass II, MD

The Hypertension Report.
Say Good Bye to High Blood Pressure.

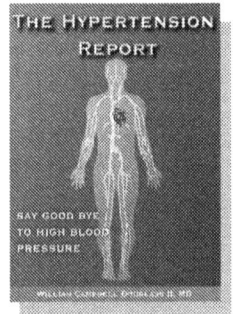

An estimated 50 million Americans have high blood pressure. Often called the "silent killer" because it may not cause symptoms until the patient has suffered serious damage to the arterial system. Diet, exercise, potassium supplements chelation therapy and practically anything but drugs is the way to go and alternatives are discussed in this report.

Grandma Bell's A To Z Guide To Healing With Herbs.

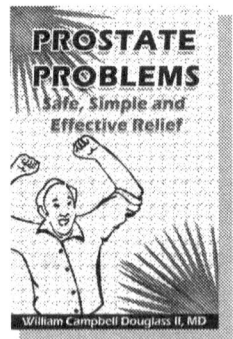

This book is all about - coming home. What I once believed to be old wives' tales - stories long destroyed by the new world of science - actually proved to be the best treatment for many of the common ailments you and I suffer through. So I put a few of them together in this book with the sincere hope that Grandma Bell's wisdom will help you recover your common sense, and take responsibility for your own health. -William Campbell Douglass II, MD

Prostate Problems:
Safe, Simple, Effective Relief for Men over 50.

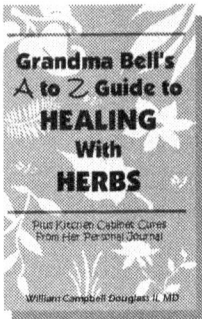

Don't be frightened into surgery or drugs you may not need. First, get the facts about prostate problems... know all your options, so you can make the best decisions. This fully documented report explains the dangers of conventional treatments, and gives you alternatives that could save you more than just money!

Color me Healthy
The Healing Powers of Colors

"He's crazy!"
"He's got to be a quack!"
"Who gave this guy his medical license?"
"He's a nut case!"

In case you're wondering, those are the reactions you'll probably get if you show your doctor this report. I know the idea of healing many common ailments simply by exposing them to colored light sounds far-fetched, but when you see the evidence, you'll agree that color is truly an amazing medical breakthrough.

When I first heard the stories, I reacted much the same way. But the evidence so convinced me, that I had to try color therapy in my practice. My results were truly amazing.

-William Campbell Douglass II, MD

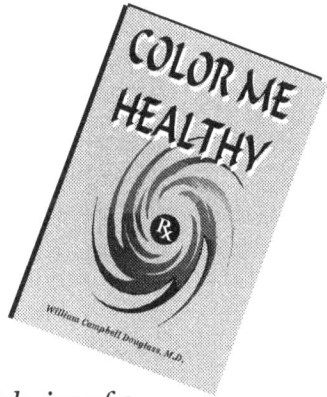

Order your complete set of Roscolene filters (choice of 3 sizes) to be used with the "Color Me Healthy" therapy. The eleven Roscolene filters are # 809, 810, 818, 826, 828, 832, 859, 861, 866, 871, and 877. The filters come with protective separator sheets between each filter. The color names and the Roscolene filter(s) used to produce that particular color, are printed on a card included with the filters and a set of instructions on how to fit them to a lamp.

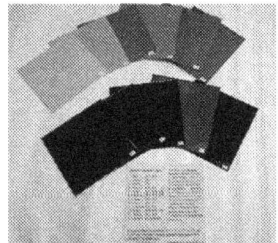

Rhino Publishing
www.rhinopublish.com

What Is Going on Here?

Peroxides are supposed to be bad for you. Free radicals and all that. But now we hear that hydrogen peroxide is good for us. Hydrogen peroxide will put extra oxygen in your blood. There's no doubt about that. Hydrogen peroxide costs pennies. So if you can get oxygen into the blood cheaply and safely, maybe cancer (which doesn't like oxygen), emphysema, AIDS, and many other terrible diseases can be treated effectively. Intravenous hydrogen peroxide rapidly relieves allergic reactions, influenza symptoms, and acute viral infections.

No one expects to live forever. But we would all like to have a George Burns finish. The prospect of finishing life in a nursing home after abandoning your tricycle in the mobile home park is not appealing. Then comes the loss of control of vital functions the ultimate humiliation. Is life supposed to be from tricycle to tricycle and diaper to diaper? You come into this world crying, but do you have to leave crying? I don't believe you do. And you won't either after you see the evidence. Sounds too good to be true, doesn't it? Read on and decide for yourself.

-William Campbell Douglass II, MD

Rhino Publishing S.A.
www.rhinopublish.com

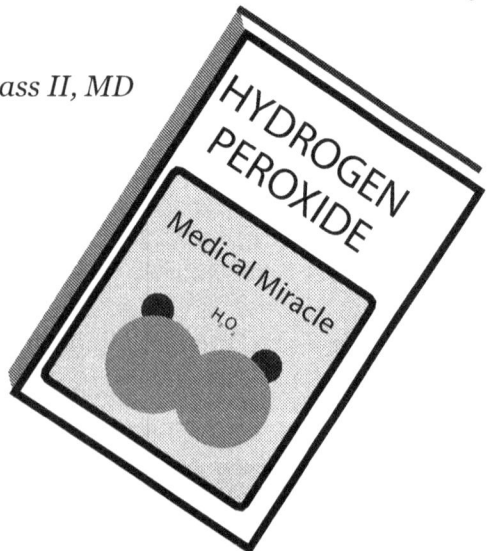

HYDROGEN PEROXIDE

Medical Miracle

H₂O

Don't drink your milk!

If you knew what we know about milk... BLEECHT! All that pasteurization, homogenization and processing is not only cooking all the nutrients right out of your favorite drink. It's also adding toxic levels of vitamin D.

This fascinating book tells the whole story about milk. How it once was nature's perfect food...how "raw," unprocessed milk can heal and boost your immune system ... why you can't buy it legally in this country anymore, and what we could do to change that.

Dr. "Douglass traveled all over the world, tasting all kinds of milk from all kinds of cows, poring over dusty research books in ancient libraries far from home, to write this light-hearted but scientifically sound book.

Rhino Publishing, S.A.
www.rhinopublish.com

The Milk Book

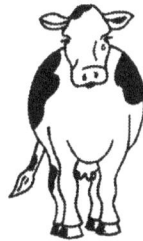

William Campbell Douglass II, MD

Eat Your Cholesterol!
Eat Meat, Drink Milk, Spread The Butter- And Live Longer!
How to Live off the Fat of the Land and Feel Great.

Americans are being saturated with anti-cholesterol propaganda. If you watch very much television, you're probably one of the millions of Americans who now has a terminal case of cholesterol phobia. The propaganda is relentless and is often designed to produce fear and loathing of this worst of all food contaminants. You never hear the food propagandists bragging about their product being fluoride-free or aluminum-free, two of our truly serious food-additive problems. But cholesterol, an essential nutrient, not proven to be harmful in any quantity, is constantly pilloried as a menace to your health. If you don't use corn oil, Fleischmann's margarine, and Egg Beaters, you're going straight to atherosclerosis hell with stroke, heart attack, and premature aging -- and so are your kids. Never feel guilty about what you eat again! Dr. Douglass shows you why red meat, eggs, and dairy products aren't the dietary demons we're told they are. But beware: This scientifically sound report goes against all the "common wisdom" about the foods you should eat. Read with an open mind.

Rhino Publishing, S.A.
www.rhinopublish.com

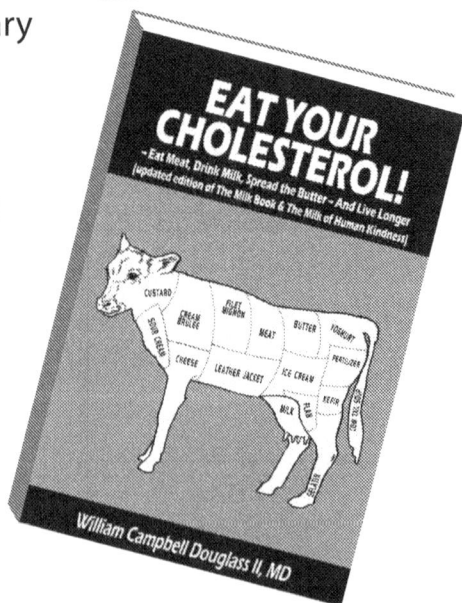

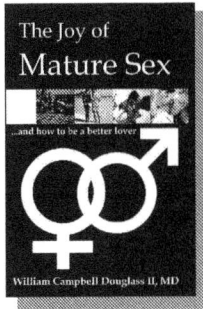

The Joy of Mature Sex and How to Be a Better Lover

Humans are very confused about what makes good sex. But I believe humans have more to offer each other than this total licentiousness common among animals. We're talking about mature sex. The kind of sex that made this country great.

Stop Aging or Slow the Process How Exercise With Oxygen Therapy (EWOT) Can Help

EWOT (pronounced ee-watt) stands for Exercise With Oxygen Therapy. This method of prolonging your life is so simple and you can do it at home at a minimal cost. When your cells don't get enough oxygen, they degenerate and die and so you degenerate and die. It's as simple as that.

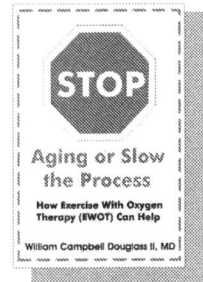

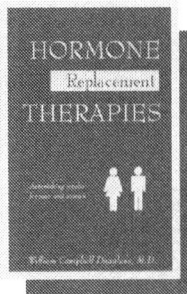

Hormone Replacement Therapies: Astonishing Results For Men And Women

It is accurate to say that when the endocrine glands start to fail, you start to die. We are facing a sea change in longevity and health in the elderly. Now, with the proper supplemental hormones, we can slow the aging process and, in many cases, reverse some of the signs and symptoms of aging.

Add 10 Years to Your Life With some "best of" Dr. Douglass' writings.

To add ten years to your life, you need to have the right attitude about health and an understanding of the health industry and what it's feeding you. Following the established line on many health issues could make you very sick or worse! Achieve dynamic health with this collection of some of the "best of" Dr. Douglass' newsletters.

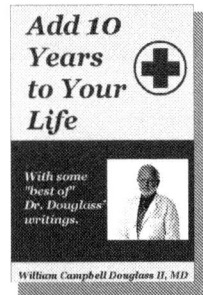

How did AIDS become one of the Greatest Biological Disasters in the History of Mankind?

GET THE FACTS

AIDS and BIOLOGICAL WARFARE covers the history of plagues from the past to today's global confrontation with AIDS, the Prince of Plagues. Completely documented *AIDS and BIOLOGICAL WARFARE* helps you make your own decisions about how to survive in a world ravaged by this horrible plague.

You will learn that AIDS is not a naturally occuring disease process as you have been led to believe, but a man-made biological nightmare that has been unleashed and is now threatening the very existence of human life on the planet.

There is a smokescreen of misinformation clouding the AIDS issue. Now, for the first time, learn the truth about the nature of the crisis our planet faces: its origin -- how AIDS is really transmited and alternatives for treatment. Find out what they are not telling you about AIDS and Biological Warfare, and how to protect yourself and your loved ones. AIDS is a serious problem worldwide, but it is no longer the major threat. You need to know the whole story. To protect yourself, you must know the truth about biological warfare.

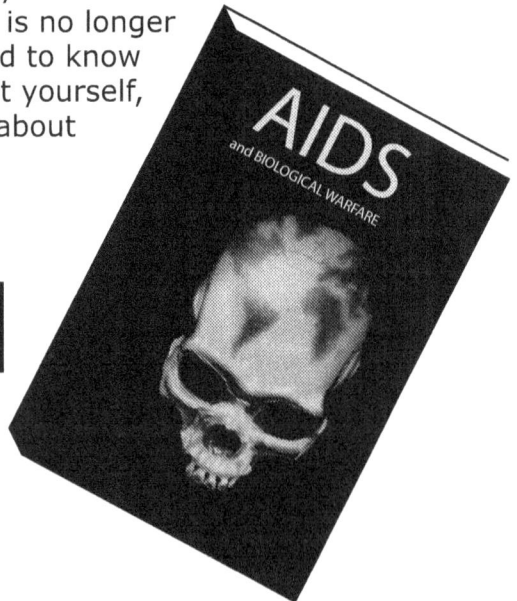

Live the Adventure!

Why would anyone in their right mind put everything they own in storage and move to Russia, of all places?! But when maverick physician Bill Douglass left a profitable medical practice in a peaceful mountaintop town to pursue "pure medical truth".... none of us who know him well was really surprised.

After All, anyone who's braved the outermost reaches of darkest Africa, the mean streets of Johannesburg and New York, and even a trip to Washington to testify before the Senate, wouldn't bat and eye at ducking behind the Iron Curtain for a little medical reconnaissance!

Enjoy this imaginative, funny, dedicated man's tales of wonder and woe as he treks through a year in St. Petersburg, working on a cure for the world's killer diseases. We promise --

YOU WON'T BE BORED!

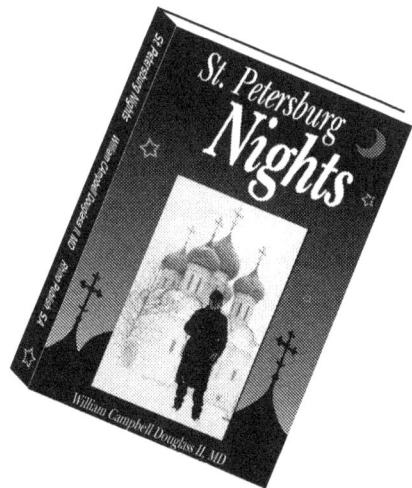

Rhino Publishing S.A.
www.rhinopublish.com

St. Petersburg Nights

William Campbell Douglass II, MD

THE SMOKER'S PARADOX
THE HEALTH BENEFITS OF TOBACCO!

The benefits of smoking tobacco have been common knowledge for centuries. From sharpening mental acuity to maintaining optimal weight, the relatively small risks of smoking have always been outweighed by the substantial improvement to mental and physical health. Hysterical attacks on tobacco notwithstanding, smokers always weigh the good against the bad and puff away or quit according to their personal preferences. Now the same anti-tobacco enterprise that has spent billions demonizing the pleasure of smoking is providing additional reasons to smoke. Alzheimer's, Parkinson's, Tourette's Syndrome, even schizophrenia and cocaine addiction are disorders that are alleviated by tobacco. Add in the still inconclusive indication that tobacco helps to prevent colon and prostate cancer and the endorsement for smoking tobacco by the medical establishment is good news for smokers and non-smokers alike. Of course the revelation that tobacco is good for you is ruined by the pharmaceutical industry's plan to substitute the natural and relatively inexpensive tobacco plant with their overpriced and ineffective nicotine substitutions. Still, when all is said and done, the positive revelations regarding tobacco are very good reasons indeed to keep lighting those cigars - but only 4 a day!

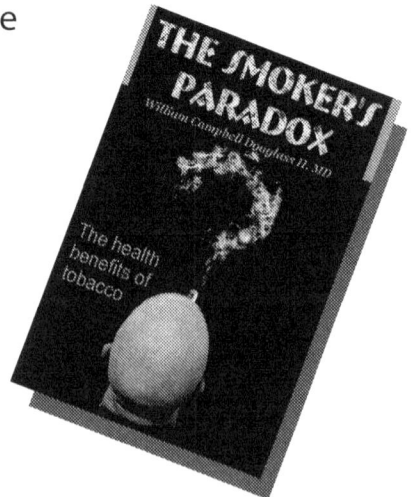

Rhino Publishing, S.A
www.rhinopublish.com

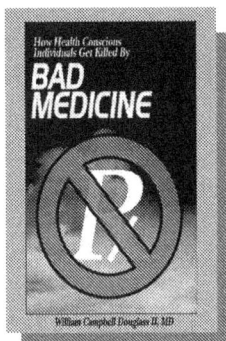

Bad Medicine
How Individuals Get Killed By Bad Medicine.

Do you really need that new prescription or that overnight stay in the hospital? In this report, Dr. Douglass reveals the common medical practices and misconceptions endangering your health. Best of all, he tells you the pointed (but very revealing!) questions your doctor prays you never ask. Interesting medical facts about popular remedies are revealed.

Dangerous Legal Drugs
The Poisons in Your Medicine Chest.

If you knew what we know about the most popular prescription and over-the-counter drugs, you'd be sick. That's why Dr. Douglass wrote this shocking report about the poisons in your medicine chest. He gives you the low-down on different categories of drugs. Everything from painkillers and cold remedies to tranquilizers and powerful cancer drugs.

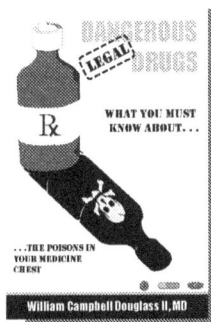

The William Campbell Douglass Letters.
Expose of Government Machinations (Vietnam War).

THE WILLIAM CAMPBELL DOUGLASS LETTERS. Dr. Douglass' Defense in 1968 Tax Case and Expose of Government Machinations during the Vietnam War.

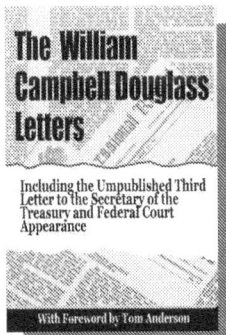

The Eagle's Feather. A Novel of International Political Intrigue.

Although The Eagle's Feather is a work of fiction set in the 1970's, it is built, as with most fiction, on a framework of plausibility and background information. This is a fiction book that could not have been written were it not for various ominous aspects, which pose a clear and present danger to the security of the United States.

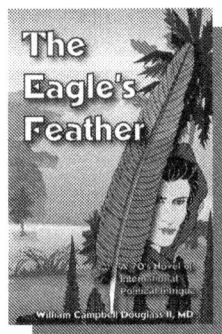

Rhino Publishing

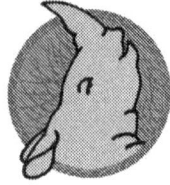

ORDER FORM

PURCHASER INFORMATION

Purchaser's Name (Please Print): _____

Shipping Address (Do not use a P.O. Box): _____

City: _____ State/Prov.: _____ Country: _____

Zip/Postal Code: _____ Telephone No.: _____ Fax No.: _____

E-Mail Address (if interested in receiving free e-Books when available): _____

CREDIT CARD INFO (CIRCLE ONE):

MASTERCARD, VISA, AMERICAN EXPRESS, DISCOVER, JCB, DINER'S CLUB, CARTE BLANCHE.

Charge my Card -> Number #: _____ Exp.: _____

*Security Code: _____ * Required for all MasterCard, Visa and American Express purchases. For your security, we require that you enter your card's verification number. The verification number is also called a CCV number. This code is the 3 digits farthest right in the signature field on the back of your VISA/MC, or the 4 digits to the right on the front of your American Express card. Your credit card statement will show **a different name than Rhino Publishing** as the vendor.

WE DO NOT share your private information, we use 3ʳᵈ party credit card processing service to process your order only.

ADDITIONAL INFORMATION

If your shipping address is not the same as your credit card billing address, please indicate your card billing address here.

_____   Type of card: _____

Name on the card

Billing Address: _____

City: _____   State/Prov.: _____   Zip/Postal Code: _____

Fax a copy of this order to:
RHINO PUBLISHING, S.A.
1-888-317-6767 or International #: + 416-352-5126

To order by mail, send your payment by first class mail only to the following address. Please include a copy of this order form. Make your check or bank drafts (NO postal money order) payable to RHINO PUBLISHING, S.A. and mail to:

Rhino Publishing, S.A.
Attention: PTY 5048
P.O. Box 025724
Miami, FL.
USA 33102

Digital E-books also available online: www.rhinopublish.com

Rhino Publishing

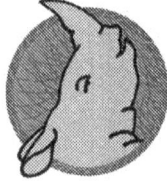

ORDER FORM

Purchaser's Name (Please Print): _____

I would like to order the following paperback book of Dr. Douglass (Alternative Medicine Books):

___	X	9962-636-04-3	Add 10 Years to Your Life. With some "best of" Dr. Douglass writings.	$13.99	$___
___	X	9962-636-07-8	AIDS and Biological Warfare. What They Are Not Telling You!	$17.99	$___
___	X	9962-636-09-4	Bad Medicine. How Individuals Get Killed By Bad Medicine.	$11.99	$___
___	X	9962-636-10-8	Color Me Healthy. The Healing Power of Colors.	$11.99	$___
___	X	9962-636 -XX-X	Color Filters for Color Me Healthy. 11 Basic Roscolene Filters for Lamps.	$21.89	$___
___	X	9962-636-15-9	Dangerous Legal Drugs. The Poisons in Your Medicine Chest.	$13.99	$___
___	X	9962-636-18-3	Dr. Douglass' Complete Guide to Better Vision. Improve eyesight naturally.	$11.99	$___
___	X	9962-636-19-1	Eat Your Cholesterol! How to Live off the Fat of the Land and Feel Great.	$11.99	$___
___	X	9962-636-12-4	Grandma Bell's A To Z Guide To Healing. Her Kitchen Cabinet Cures.	$14.99	$___
___	X	9962-636-22-1	Hormone Replacement Therapies. Astonishing Results For Men & Women	$11.99	$___
___	X	9962-636-25-6	Hydrogen Peroxide: One of the Most Underused Medical Miracle.	$15.99	$___
___	X	9962-636-27-2	Into the Light. New Edition with Blood Irradiation Instrument Instructions.	$19.99	$___
___	X	9962-636-54-X	Milk Book. The Classic on the Nutrition of Milk and How to Benefit from it.	$17.99	$___

___ X	9962-636-00-0	Painful Dilemma - Patients in Pain - People in Prison.	$17.99 $ ___
___ X	9962-636-32-9	Prostate Problems. Safe, Simple, Effective Relief for Men over 50.	$11.99 $ ___
___ X	9962-636-34-5	St. Petersburg Nights. Enlightening Story of Life and Science in Russia.	$17.99 $ ___
___ X	9962-636-37-X	Stop Aging or Slow the Process. Exercise With Oxygen Therapy Can Help.	$11.99 $ ___
___ X	9962-636-60-4	The Hypertension Report. Say Good Bye to High Blood Pressure.	$11.99 $ ___
___ X	9962-636-48-5	The Joy of Mature Sex and How to Be a Better Lover...	$13.99 $ ___
___ X	9962-636-43-4	The Smoker's Paradox: Health Benefits of Tobacco.	$14.99 $ ___

Political Books:

___ X	9962-636-40-X	The Eagle's Feather. A 70's Novel of International Political Intrigue.	$15.99 $ ___
___ X	9962-636-46-9	The W. C. D. Letters. Expose of Government Machinations (Vietnam War).	$11.99 $ ___
		SUB-TOTAL:	$ ___

ADD $5.00 HANDLING FOR YOUR ORDER: $ 5.00 $ 5.00

___ X ADD $2.50 SHIPPING FOR EACH ITEM ON ORDER: $ 2.50 $ ___

NOTE THAT THE MINIMUM SHIPPING AND HANDLING IS $7.50 FOR 1 BOOK ($5.00 + $2.50)

For order shipped outside the US, add $5.00 per item

___ X ADD $5.00 S. & H. OR EACH ITEM ON ORDER (INTERNATIONAL ORDERS ONLY) $ 5.00 $ ___

Allow up to 21 days for delivery (we will call you about back orders if any)

TOTAL: $ ___

Fax a copy of this order to: 1-888-317-6767 or Int'l + 416-352-5126
or mail to: Rhino Publishing, S.A. Attention: PTY 5048 P.O. Box 025724, Miami, FL., 33102 USA
Digital E-books also available online: www.rhinopublish.com

www.ingramcontent.com/pod-product-compliance
Lightning Source LLC
Chambersburg PA
CBHW032052020426
42335CB00011B/309